P9-BTN-652

CONTENTS

Part 1   An Overview

Part 2   Problems of Childhood and Adolescence

85174

PREVENTIVE PSYCHIATRY

*Early Intervention and
Situational Crisis Management*

EDITED BY

Samuel C. Klagsbrun, MD
Gilbert W. Kliman, MD
Elizabeth J. Clark, PhD, ACSW
Austin H. Kutscher, DDS
Robert DeBellis, MD
Carole A. Lambert, RN

The Charles Press, Publishers
Philadelphia

The Charles Press, Publishers
Post Office Box 15715
Philadelphia, Pennsylvania
19103

Library of Congress Catalog Card Number: 88-0663414

ISBN 0-914783-28-9 (hardbound)
ISBN 0-914783-29-7 (softbound)

Managing Editor: Sanford Robinson
Editorial Assistant: Audrey Bedics
Compositor: Cage Graphic Arts, Inc.
Designed by Sanford Robinson
Printed by Princeton University Press

5 4 3 2 1

Chapter 7, "Facilitation of Mourning during Childhood," by Gilbert Kliman, was reprinted with permission from Gerber I, Weiner A, Kutscher AH, et al (eds): *Perspectives on Bereavement.* © 1979 by Arno Press, Inc.

Special thanks to Lawrence McFadden and Reba Bartash for their unflagging patience and professionalism.

Part 4 Problems of Health Care Professionals

EDITORS

Samuel C. Klagsbrun, MD
Associate Clinical Professor of Psychiatry, College of Physicians and Surgeons, Columbia University, New York, New York; Director, Four Winds Hospital, Katonah, New York

Gilbert W. Kliman, MD
Director, Preventive Psychiatry Services, St. Mary's Hospital and Medical Center, San Francisco, California; Founder and Edtior, *The Journal of Preventive Psychiatry;* Founder, Center for Preventive Psychiatry, White Plains and Yonkers, New York

Elizabeth J. Clark, ACSW, PhD
Assistant Professor, Department of Health Professions, Montclair State College, Upper Montclair, New Jersey

Austin H. Kutscher, DDS
President, The Foundation of Thanatology, New York, New York; Professor of Dentistry (in Psychiatry), Department of Psychiatry, College of Physicians and Surgeons, Columbia University, New York, New York

Robert DeBellis, MD
Assistant Professor of Clinical Medicine (Oncology), College of Physicians and Surgeons, Columbia University, New York, New York

Carole A. Lambert, RN
Psychiatric Nurse Clinician, Jewish Home for the Aged, Bronx, New York

CONTRIBUTORS

Virginia W. Barrett, RN, MEd
Community Health Nursing Consultant, Columbia University Center for Geriatrics and Gerontology, The Faculty of Medicine of Columbia University; New York State Office of Mental Health, New York, NY

D. Peter Birkett, MD
Associate Research Scientist, Department of Psychiatry, Columbia University Center for Geriatrics and Gerontology, The Faculty of Medicine of Columbia University, New York, NY; Medical Director, Riverside Nursing Home, Suffern, NY

Paul M. Brinich, PhD
Director, Childhood Loss Program; Assistant Professor of Child Therapy, University Hospitals of Cleveland, OH

Elizabeth J. Clark, ACSW, PhD
Assistant Professor, Department of Health Professions, Montclair State College, Upper Montclair, NJ

Francine Cournos, MD
Assistant Clinical Professor of Psychiatry, College of Physicians and Surgeons, Columbia University, New York, NY

Alice D. Cullinan, PhD
Middletown Psychiatric Center, Middletown, NY

A. Elaine Cummings, RN
Formerly Educational Director, St. Francis Center, Washington, DC

Joel S. Delfiner, MD
Chief, Neuromuscular Division, Department of Neurology; Director, Muscular Dystrophy Clinic, Nassau County Medical Center, East Meadow, NY

Tamara Ferguson, PhD
Adjunct Associate Professor of Sociology in Psychiatry, Department of Psychiatry, Wayne State University, Detroit, MI

Frances K. Forstenzer, LCSW
Private Practice; Center for Living, Baltimore, MD

Sandra S. Fox, PhD, ACSW
Director, The Good Grief Program, Boston, MA

Alicia J. Goral, RN, MSN
Psychiatric Nurse Instructor, Rockford Memorial School, Rockford, IL

Dorothea Hays, EdD, RN
Professor (graduate program), Adelphi University, School of Nursing, Garden City, NY

Sherry E. Johnson, RN, PhD
Private Practice, Hingham, MA

Diane Kramer, CSW
Doctoral Candidate, Adelphi University School of Social Work; Private Practice, Psychotherapist and Bereavement Consultant, Garden City, NY

Claire F. Leach, MSS
Medical Social Worker, Nassau County Medical Center, East Meadow, NY

Stephen Lubowe, MS
Independent Scholar, The Foundation of Thanatology, New York, NY

Helen Miles, BS, RN, ASPO
Director (Ret'd), Nursing and Health Services, Graduate Program, Adelphi University School of Nursing, Garden City, NY

Avtandil A. Papiasvili, MD
Institute of Psychiatry, Department of Psychiatry, Cornell University Medical College, Westchester Division; The New York Hospital, White Plains, NY

June C. Penney, PhD
Assistant Professor and Chairman, Curriculum Committee on Death and Dying, Dalhousie Medical School, Department of anatomy/Faculty of Medicine, Halifax, Nova Scotia, Canada

Marilyn M. Rawnsley, DNSc
Visiting Professor, Department of Nursing Education, Teachers College, Columbia University, New York, NY

David P. Roye, Jr., MD
Assistant Professor of Clinical Orthopedic Surgery, College of Physicians and Surgeons, Columbia University, New York, NY

Diane M. Ryerson, MS, ACSW
Coordinator of Consultation and Education, and Director of ASAP, South Virgin Mental Health Center, Inc., Lynhurst and Hackensack, NJ

Daniel J. Schaefer
Author and Funeral Director, Brooklyn, NY

Irene B. Seeland, MD
Assistant Clinical Professor of Psychiatry, New York University School of Medicine; Attending Psychiatrist, Goldwater Memorial Hospital, New York, NY

Florence Selder, RN, PhD
Associate Professor, Urban Research Center, University of Wisconsin, Milwaukee; Clinical Associate Professor, The Midwest Center for Human Sciences, Milwaukee, WI

Sally K. Severino, MD
Assistant Professor of Psychiatry, Department of Psychiatry, Mew York Hospital-Cornell Medical Center; Collaborating Psychoanalyst, Columbia University, Center for Psychoanalytic Training and Research, New York, NY

William J. Sobotor
Assistant Professor and Instructor, Radiation Therapy Technicians Program, College of Health Related Professions, State University of New York, Syracuse, NY

Jack M. Stack, MD
Family Health Research, Education and Services Institute, Alma, MI

Robert G. Stevenson, EdD
Instructor of Death Education Programs of River Dell High School; Fairleigh Dickinson and Bergen Community College, NJ; Co-Chairperson, Columbia University Seminar on Death, Columbia University, New York, NY

William Weiner, ACSW
Psychotherapist, Private Practice; Department of Social Work Services, Bronx Veterans Administration Hospital, Bronx, NY

Rev. William A. Wendt, STD
Executive Director, St. Francis Center, Washington, DC

Arthur B. Zelman, MD
Medical Director, Center for Preventive Psychiatry, White Plains, NY

PREFACE

This book is based on the premise that many emotional illnesses can be prevented or at least ameliorated by early intervention and appropriate treatment during the incipient stages of the disorder. Put differently, by recognizing high-risk situations that are likely to give rise to mental illness in the future, it is possible to apply preventive measures at the time and head off subsequent problems.

This concept focused initially on young children who had experienced a critical loss, particularly the death of a parent. The underlying goal was to facilitate mourning as a means of averting the well-known sequelae of bereavement in childhood (for example, depression so commonly observed among orphans in later years). It soon became evident that a preventive approach could also be utilized successfully in dealing with object loss at any age, not only in children. Indeed, the importance of object loss in the pathogenesis of emotional illnesses is now well established, and the management of loss and bereavement has become a cornerstone of preventive psychiatry, as explained throughout this book.

Also in the sphere of preventive psychiatry is crisis intervention, especially in situational crises. Traumatic events such as adolescent suicide, rape, crime victimization, life-threatening illness, sudden death in the family, and similar crises cause severe stress for victims and their families. The long-term effects of these situational crises may be avoided or controlled by preventive therapeutic measures. In fact, many believe that preventive psychiatry has its widest application in this particular area. In keeping with the expanded version of the term "crisis" to include developmental and maturational changes as well as situational crisis, the scope of prevention has become even broader. In any case, the concept that prompt, preventive intervention can halt or diminish the severity of emotional illness has brought forth many exciting prospects.

Written and edited by the leading workers in the field, *Preventive Psychiatry* explores the principles and actual practices of preventive psychiatry, providing a clear view of current thinking and future directions. We believe that the book will be of great interest to psychiatrists and other mental health professionals, including social workers, nurses, psychologists, clergy, guidance counsellors, occupational therapists, and others involved in loss management and crisis intervention.

ACKNOWLEDGMENT

The editors wish to acknowledge the support and encouragement of the Foundation of Thanatology in the preparation of this volume. All royalties from the sale of this book are assigned to the Foundation of Thanatology, a tax exempt, not for profit, public scientific and educational foundation.

Thanatology, a new subspecialty of medicine, is involved in scientific and humanistic inquiries and the application of the knowledge derived therefrom to the subjects of the psychological aspects of dying; reactions to loss, death, and grief; and recovery from bereavement.

PART 1

An Overview

1

Preventive Psychiatry and Object Loss:
Development of a Preventive Clinic

Arthur B. Zelman

The idea of prevention in psychiatry is borrowed from the public-health approach to medicine. In this approach three levels of prevention are identified; primary, secondary and tertiary. Primary prevention involves the reduction of incidence of an illness, secondary prevention attempts to reduce the illness' duration and severity, and tertiary prevention involves minimization of impairment and enhancement of compensatory mechanisms (i.e., rehabilitation).

Fundamental to the concept of prevention is an understanding of the etiology of the disorder. By recognizing the causes of an illness, it becomes possible, theoretically at least, to prevent the illness by eliminating or attenuating the causative factors.

Two major precepts regarding the possible etiology of mental illness emerged in the early 20th century, which later formed the foundations for preventive psychiatry. First, it became evident that the experiences of childhood shape the development of the adult, or, as Wordsworth expressed it, "The child is father of the man." Thus, a key etiological factor in the development of adult psychopathology is that of unresolved emotional stresses and strains of childhood, particularly those associated with loss. By attending to a child's emotional problems at the time of the loss, prevention of lifelong adult disorders might be achieved.

A second etiological tenet recognized about the same time was the importance of experiences compared to biological (hereditary) factors in determining behavior. In other terms, social and environmental forces play a significant role in personality formation and structure.

Two developments at the turn of the 20th century focused attention on these two ideas. The first was the progressive social-welfare movement, which, among other things, promulgated child labor laws out of its concern for the powerless in society. From this tradition emerged the mental hygiene movement headed by Clifford Beers.

The second development was the advent in American philosophy of positivism and pragmatism. In the tradition of John Locke's *tabula rasa* — the child's mind as a blank slate upon which his experiences would be inscribed — these theories, particularly John Dewey's, led to a focus on the importance of education. Just as a proper positivist-inspired education could lead to a well educated and highly developed human being, the assumption was that poor education would lead to the opposite. This point of view helped spur interest in learning theory and behavior in the fields of academic and clinical psychology. The ideas of Dewey and James also influenced Adolph Meyer, one of the more influential figures in American psychiatry during the first half of the 20th century. Working and writing at the same time as Freud, Meyer emphasized the relevance of psychological and social factors to the understanding of psychopathology.

These currents of early 20th-century thought were contemporaneous with the early evolution of psychoanalytic thinking. Freud's theory of infantile sexuality provided a framework for exploring the relationship of early childhood development to the normal and abnormal psychology of the adult. In his "Three Essays on Sexuality," Freud suggested a link between childhood sexuality, i.e., early childhood development, and adult psychopathology, especially neuroses and sexual disorders. He also alluded to early experience as influencing the sexuality of the child. Moreover, his work with the father of Little Hans implied a belief in the possibility of early intervention.

On the one hand, insofar as he based much of his theory of sexuality on bisexuality and instinct theory and later on the inevitable demands made upon the individual by culture, Freud's theory of the etiology of mental illness discouraged the idea of prevention.

Freud's shifting attitude toward female hysteria had mixed implications for prevention. His early view that his female patients' accounts of molestation in childhood were reality-based, while much resisted by his culture, nevertheless would have provided food for preventive thought. Instead, as has recently been widely discussed in the lay as well as professional literature, he altered his position to the more "biologically" oriented and—from a preventive point of view — more pessimistic notion that these patients' material reflected wish-driven fantasies, not realities.

The concept of object loss as applied to emphasis on early childhood on the one hand and to the social environment on the other, proved crucial for a psychoanalytic theory of prevention. In his essay "Mourning and Melancholia," Freud stressed the importance of object loss as a precipitant of both. In 1946, following up on this theoretical importance of object loss, René Spitz described the syndrome of anaclitic depression resulting from infants' loss of their mothers during the second half of the first year of life. Rapid reversal of symptoms recurred following the therapeutic "measure" of restoration to the children of their mothers. This proved a watershed study. In the 1940s and 1950s many others, including A. Freud, Burlingham, Prugh, Robertson and Bowlby, studied infants and young children separated from their parents. As with Spitz's work, opportunities for preventive interventions were identified.

For example, studies of children hospitalized for medical problems led to changes in hospital procedures, such as allowing the parent to remain with the child and preparation of the child through play and age-appropriate explanations of planned medical procedures.

Freud made use of the comparison between mourning and depression and develop his concept of the ego and its relationship to the superego. He states, in the same essay, that the loss of the libidinal, i.e., primary, object in childhood leads to "an identification of the ego with the abandoned object. Thus the shadow of the object falls upon the ego and the latter can henceforth be judged by a special agency as though it were an object, the forsaken object" (*ibid*, p. 249). The agency referred to is conscience or the superego. Freud alludes to Abraham's concept of depression as relating to identification or incorporation of the lost object in the oral phase. Here he is implying that object loss during the oral phase, i.e., the first year or so, may be fateful because of the superego's consequent critical attitude toward the abandoning object now installed in the ego.

Since, according to Freud's theory, conscience, or the superego, only develops later in the course of the resolution of the Oedipal complex, the two phenomena — setting up the "lost" object in the ego, and the attack on the object in the ego — seem to be out of phase.

Several questions pertinent to prevention were thus raised by Freud's use of object loss to illuminate melancholia. Who or what is the nature of the object such that its loss would have serious consequences? What exactly constitutes "loss" of an object? What are the different effects of object loss at different ages and stages of development? At what age, for example, will object loss be more likely to result in a propensity for melancholia, or precipitate melancholia, or merely result in the process of mourning?

In a 1923 paper entitled "The Ego and the Id," Freud stated that "the character of the ego is a precipitate of abandoned object-cathexis." He was again referring to the mechanism of identification with the lost object; this time, however, using it to explain not only the illness of melancholia but the normal development of the ego. Hence, he had taken the concept of object loss and used it as a cornerstone of his structural theory of the mind.

Freud's structural theory, in particular his focus on the concept of the ego, was to begin a line of thinking which would take classical psychoanalysis away from the preventive dead-end of his earlier notions. Following this lead, the development during the next three decades of ego psychology (especially Hartmann's idea of the autonomous functions of the ego) helped to weaken the primacy of instinct theory. This theoretical development cleared the way for many psychoanalysts to view with greater interest the idea of prevention.

Freud's emphasis in "Mourning and Melancholia" on narcissistic object choice combined with the idea of "traumatic experiences in connection with the object" implied that the key to understanding depression might be found in the young child's relations to objects. After the publication of "The Ego and the Id" early object relations could be implicated in broader issues of development, both normal and abnormal.

In "Mourning and Melancholia" Freud also pointed out that occasions which enhance ambivalence and might therefore give rise to depression included "all those situations of being slighted, neglected or disappointed." Hence, it was not only the loss of an object that was important but the quality of the relationship. By 1940, Freud had concluded that the original mother–child relationship would remain a prototype of the child's later love relations. Hence, the way was open to the study of the content and quality of this relationship, in addition to its loss, as a means of understanding adult pathology. The clinical work of Spitz, Mahler and Fraiberg, the experimental work of Emde, and the ethological approach of Bowlby and Ainsworth among many others all reflect the growing interest in the early parent–child relationship as a basis for primary and secondary preventive interventions.

Interest in bereavement also took another direction with implications for prevention. In 1944 Erich Lindemann published his classic study describing the syndrome of acute grief. Included in this study were relatives of people who had died in a fire. Lindemann briefly described the work of mourning that the survivors would have to do, with or without help, to make an adequate adjustment. This study, with its emphasis on the facilitation of mourning, became a model for what was later to be called crisis intervention.

Concepts such as stress-response, adaptation, homeostasis, and mastery were quickly woven into a theory whereby early intervention could maximize coping and even growth in response to a sudden stress or loss. "Early intervention" thus acquired a second meaning. It now referred to a swift response following a stressful event, as opposed to help provided early in a child's development. Both kinds of intervention could be viewed, however, as constituting primary or secondary prevention, depending on whether illness was or was not already present.

In summary, the study of bereavement and development of the concept of object loss helped to provide a basis for preventive interrenetion.

THE CENTER FOR PREVENTIVE PSYCHIATRY*

How is preventive psychiatry actually implemented in practice and is it an effective approach? The experience of the Center for Preventive Psychiatry, described in the following pages, offers some insight into these questions.

The Center for Preventive Psychiatry is a preventively oriented public mental-health clinic located in White Plains and Yonkers, New York. Founded in 1965 by Dr. Gilbert Kliman, its initial focus was on the study and treatment of children's reactions to object loss. Within a short time, however, this interest in childhood bereavement came to function as the common point of departure for the two kinds of intervention discussed above, namely, early childhood intervention and situational crisis intervention.

The background of the Center's work in childhood bereavement is discussed in Chapter 7.

Early Childhood Services

The first discrete service to be developed at the Center was a therapeutic nursery for children under six years of age. Although initially designed to provide brief intervention for bereaved children who may or may not have been symptomatic (i.e., primary prevention), not many such children were referred. Instead, most referrals concerned children who were already symptomatic (secondary intervention). Concurrently, a survey conducted revealed that there were 3,000 preschool children in the Center's catchment area who were in need of treatment, almost none of whom were being served, and that it was children from this group who were being referred.

The Cornerstone Therapeutic Nursery was originally conceived by Dr. Kliman as an "analytic public health experiment." A child psychoanalyst was present in the therapeutic classroom and treated each child in turn in the presence of the teachers and other children. It was hoped that maximal efficiency of the psychoanalyst's time could be made in this way.

By 1977, 65% of the clinic's patients, compared to 7% of the local population at large, were impoverished. Hence, the Center was inadvertently given the opportunity to develop and provide early interventions to an impoverished sub-population in which epidemiological research had previously shown higher-than-average rates of pathology.

Included among these services was a modality based on the work of Augusta Alpert, initially referred to as educational psychotherapy. "Working with children suffering from pathological fixations due to maternal deprivation, Alpert found that when children 2 to 5 years old were given the opportunity to regress . . . they were sometimes receptive to. . . . restitutive mothering provided by their therapist." The Center instituted a training program led by childhood educators Doris Ronald and Dr. Myron Stein to enable them to employ a kind of "corrective object-relations" therapy for children thought not ready or able to utilize an interpretive modality.

At the same time, the Center provided training in child psychoanalytic psychotherapy and child psychoanalysis. This program provided psychotherapy for those children deemed developmentally advanced enough to benefit from an interpretive modality. This group included a number of children from impoverished and multi-problem families, a group not generally thought to be amenable to interpretive treatment.

In the tradition of Caplan's consultative model of prevention, the Center's early childhood intervention service also provided consultation (as well as on-site) treatment to day-care centers, nursery schools and Head Start programs.

Another offshoot of the early childhood approach was a focus on high-risk children and their families. Following an earlier pilot study, the Center, in 1978, received N.I.M.H. funding for a four year research and demonstration project to study the effects of short term intervention on children entering foster care. More recently, other high-risk groups of children have received attention. For example, consultation and on-site treatment of children and

mothers were provided to a spouse abuse shelter. Currently, consultation and
on-site intervention with incarcerated mothers and children is being provided
at a local correctional institution. The Center is also funded to provide treatment to the preschool children of mentally ill parents as well as to homeless
children and their families.

Early Intervention in Situational Crisis

One of the observations made at the Center and elsewhere in the course of
work with bereaved children was that the child's capacity to deal successfully
with the loss of a parent or sibling depended, in part, on the surviving parent's
ability to mourn. Interest in adult mourning was additionally stimulated by
studies suggesting increased rates of morbidity and mortality in bereaved
spouses. Hence, in the late 1960s the Center's Situational Crisis Service,
directed by Ann Kliman, was formed. Its purpose was to help children, adults
and families who had suffered recent bereavement or other losses or situational
stresses. Such stresses might include diagnosis of a serious illness, sudden loss
of a body part or function due to accident or illness, birth of a defective child,
loss of a job, loss of a home, move from one city or region to another, and
crime victimization.

As with the early childhood intervention service, the situational crisis service provided consultation to other agencies, and even communities. An
example of the latter was consultation provided to the community of Corning,
New York following a flood in 1972. Among other observations made was that
of an increased post-flood auto accident rate which, following the intervention,
fell below the pre-disaster baseline. This consultation was a precursor of the
larger intervention made by Kai Ericson and others following the Buffalo Creek
disaster. More typically, the Center's Situational Crisis Service provides consultation to schools, churches, and other organizations, concerning single and
multiple bereavements, suicide and homicide post-vention, separation and
divorce, and crime victimization, particularly rape. Recently consultation was
provided to a division of a large company which had undergone, in quick
succession, two changes of ownership and was expecting another, leaving the
division's fate in question for many months. The consultation was requested
by the division's employee safety committee, who feared an increase in on-the-
job accidents due to increased worker anxiety.

The two kinds of early intervention sometimes reconverge. A notable
example involved a day-care center at which multiple incidents of sexual abuse
were alleged to have occurred. Many Center clinicians from both early-
intervention services collaborated to provide consultation for Child Protective
Services staff, and group and individual interventions for parents and children.
One of the outcomes of this intervention was the successful persecution of the
perpetrators based in large part on the testimony of several of the children
whose families had participated in the consultations.

In summary, the preventive clinic described here has undergone parallel development with psychoanalytically-informed preventive theory. Both theory and practice have evolved from a focus on bereavement and object loss to a broader and still expanding understanding of opportunities for prevention.

REFERENCES

Alpert, A. 1959. "Reversibility of Pathological Fixations Associated with Maternal Deprivation in Infancy." *The Psychoanalytic Study of the Child*, 19:169-185.

Caplan, G. 1964. Principles of Preventive Psychiatry. New York: Basie Books.

Freud, S. 1953. "The Ego and the Id." *Complete Psychological Works of Sigmund Freud, Standard Edition*, vol. 19. London: Hogarth Press.

Freud, S. 1948. "Mourning and Melancholia." *Collected Papers*, vol. 4. London: Hogarth Press.

Freud, S. 1953. "Three Essays on the Theory of Sexuality," of the *Complete Psychological Works of Sigmund Freud, Standard Edition*, vol. 7. London: Hogarth Press.

Hartmann, H. 1958. *Ego Psychology and the Problem of Adaptation*. London: Image.

Kliman, A.S. 1976. "The Corning Project: Psychological First Aid Following a Natural Disaster." H. Parad, H. Resnik, L. parad, eds. In *Emergency and Disaster Management: A Mental Health Source Book. Philadelphia: Charles Press.*

Kliman, G. W. 1975. "Analyst in the Nursery: An Experimental Application of Child Analytic Techniques in a Therapeutic Nursery School: The Cornerstone Method." *The Psychoanalytic Study of the Child*, vol. 30.

Kliman, G. et al. 1982. *Preventive Mental Health Services for Children Entering Foster-Home Care: An Assessment.* White Plains, NY: Center for Preventive Psychiatry.

Lindemann, E. 1944. "Symptomatology and Management of Acute Grief. *American Journal of Psychiatry*, 101:141–148.

Rhodes, R. and A. Zelman. 1986. *An Ongoing Multi-family Group in a Women's Shelter.* American journal of Orthopsychiatry, 56:Jan.

Spitz, R. 1965. *The First Year of Life.* New York: International Universities Press.

Zelman, A. 1980. *Early Childhood Psychotherapy: Its Role in Prevention.* White Plains, NY: Center for Preventive Psychiatry.

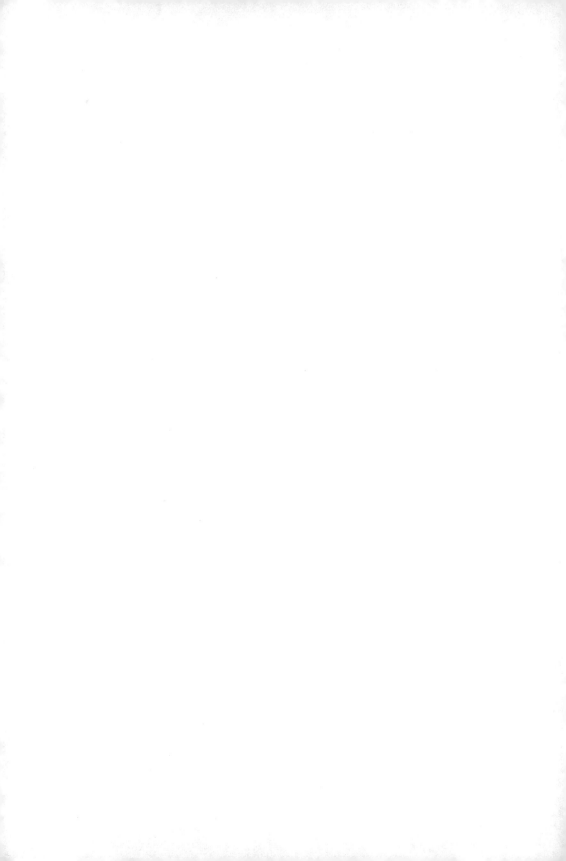

2

Learning to Grow Through Loss:

A Focus for Preventive Mental Health Services

Marilyn M. Rawnsley

Once, in a powerful and prosperous land, the citizens were roused from lethargy by the visions of their young people, who challenged why things were the way they were. And the young people, being naive and full of energy and hope, dreamed that they could change the world. Their youthful enthusiasm for their conviction was contagious; their passion for justice was compelling. Soon orators from the ruling class began to speak about equal opportunity and equal rights to ensure everyone a share in the richness of the country. Freedom itself was not a new idea in this nation, but the notion of extending it to include every citizen, regardless of age, color, sex, physical handicap, or even mental illness, incited a social revolution. There were struggles and setbacks eventually but, decrees went forth throughout the land to achieve these goals. Among other changes, sweeping reforms were attempted in the antiquated mental-health system. It seemed a brave beginning. But a long and unpopular war in a far-away country drained the youth of their passion for their homeland and destroyed their faith in its rulers. Violence seething within the society erupted, killing some of the dreamers and, with them, the dream.

● ● ●

For some of us who were educated in the 1960s, the efforts to reform the dehumanizing mental health system are synonymous with the social conscience of those times. Others see the passage, in 1963, of the Federal Community Mental Health Act, which funded the construction and staffing of community mental health centers, as a less than successful attempt to reduce the high cost of care of the mentally ill. Regardless of one's perspective or politics, most people will concede that the community mental health movement, at the least, served as a catalyst to promote public awareness not only of the problems of mental illness, but of the mental health needs of the larger population. Concepts of stress and crisis lost their pejorative connotations as issues that reflected some characterological flaw; instead they became accepted as conditions that are common to us all. In particular, the concept of crisis as described by Caplan (1964) was expanded to include developmental or maturational change, as well as situational dilemmas and loss. This expansion of the concept opened the field of preventive psychiatry beyond medicine and gave rise to a cadre of interdisciplinary mental health professionals, such as social workers, nurses, psychologists, clergy, guidance counselors, and occupational and recreational therapists, whose education and practice incorporated principles of crisis theory and crisis intervention.

Despite this apparent convergence of professionals into the arena of the crisis model as a schematic for assessment and treatment, a common conceptual core for mental health research and practice remains unclarified. The lack of such a core is an important consideration when designing preventive mental health services. If mental health is defined as the absence of signs and symptoms of pathology, then services are directed toward secondary and tertiary levels of prevention in an attempt to restore prior functioning and reduce the residual effects of illness. If mental health is perceived merely as a mirror image of mental illness, instead of as a state of being in itself, then preventive efforts necessarily focus on remediation rather than on growth.

The idealism of the 1960s created illusions of community. The social community that would provide competent care for the de-institutionalized mentally ill, as well as for persons in acute crisis, was a dream of liberal humanists. The intellectual community that would link disparate disciplines into a science of mental health was a dream of philosopher-statespersons. In reality, a body of knowledge about mental health that identifies constructs and principles from which to generate hypotheses that can be empirically tested, as well as evaluated in practice, has not been established.

If a science of mental health were to be formulated, it would include several theoretical perspectives. In this chapter, I explain a conceptual focus on loss as one perspective for the development of theories relevant to preventive mental health.

A premise basic to this perspective is that mental health involves the capacity to consider one's experience both as unique to the self and as expressions of, or variations on, the common human theme. Loss is an example of a phenomenon that is central to the human condition, yet one that each of us perceives as a personal encounter with unwanted change. Each encounter with unwanted change incorporates a dimension of potential for increasing complexity or growth. Usually, although this is less widely recognized, these occurrences of unwanted change are also vehicles for growth for those who are associated with the person who experiences it directly.

This opportunity to learn from the loss experience of others is critical to true primary preention. Identification with the loss of others can be constructively directed to strengthening one's capacity for mental health in the absence of direct threats to one's well-being. Moreover, there are prototypes of the experience of loss that are common to all of us and to which we can relate the events that others are experiencing.

CONCEPTUAL FRAMEWORK

Universal conflict situations, as described by Mann (1973:27), are four behavioral patterns that express "all the ways that humans experience loss." These situations are postulated as behavioral responses to anxiety, arising out of the attempt to master the ambivalence felt during the maturational process of separation–individuation. Mastery of this ambivalence is said to lead to a sense of control of self in relation to the external world. Separation and loss are recurring life themes; thus, threats to this sense of control are ongoing (Mann 1973, Mann and Goldman 1982).

The process of separation–individuation which begins in the early months of life, and which dominates pre-oedipal development, "reverberates throughout the life cycle" (Mahler, Bergman, and Pine 1975:3) and is never totally resolved. This developmental process, through which the self establishes its relationship to the external world, is said to be a universal lifelong phenomenon associated with biopsychosocial change as well as with object loss. Therefore, both maturational and situational crises evoke the conflict patterns that are characteristics of an individual's early behavioral responses to the anxiety of separation–individuation.

The appropriateness of this interpretation to preventive mental health seems apparent. If these proposed conflict situations can be demonstrated as responses to universal experience, then this conceptual perspective not only provides a framework for helping individuals to grow through their own losses, but also has implications for enhancing the mental health of others. Through the judicious use of vicarious learning that connects to the common human theme of separation and loss, individuals can recognize their own conflict patterns and identify strategies that promote mental health.

The four universal situations or behavioral response patterns to loss are as follows:

> **Activity versus passivity**   ". . . the degree of felt inner freedom, or lack of it, to pursue one's wishes or needs or aims with appropriate aggressiveness" (Mann 1973:28).
> **Adequate versus dimished self-esteem**   The discrepancy between the wishful concept of the self and self-representation (Parens 1971).
> **Unresolved or delayed grief**   Object losses that are not fully mourned but are translated symbolically in the ego (Fenichel 1945, Gaylin 1968, Winnicott 1965).
> **Independence versus dependence**   Lifelong tension between the wish to be independent and the temptation to regress to an earlier dependent state (Mann and Goldman 1982).

The literature on object-relations theory provides theoretical support for the origin and development of these conflict situations. For example, Parens (1971:124) placed the beginning of psychological dependence in the initial experience of separation anxiety when the narcissistic infant becomes aware that he or she is not omnipotent but is "nigh-totally sustained from without."

The activity–passivity conflict has both cognitive and affective dimensions. The studies of Weissman, Wordin, and Sobel (1980) indicate that effective conflict resolution is associated with active problem-solving strategies, whereas feelings of isolation, victimization, and suppressed emotion are associated with passive avoidance behaviors.

Self-esteem is, of course, the degree of regard one has for oneself. Adequate self-esteem is characterized by feelings of self-worth and value and by confidence in one's actions (Fitts 1965). Diminished self-esteem is reflected in attitudes of self-doubt, personal undesirability, and unhappiness (Fitts 1965, Mann 1943).

Experiences with loss begin when the infant is required to give up significant objects. Winnicott (1965), building on Klein's (1940) substantive work on the emotional life of infants, describes this developmental process as the depressive position, a normal and essential component of growth during the weaning stage. Successful mastery of this early loss is equated with later responses of grief and sadness in the normal mourning process (Gaylin 1968). Failure to achieve mastery results, however, in response patterns of unresolved or delayed grief.

RESEARCH AND PRACTICE IMPLICATIONS

Despite the theoretical support for the construct of universal conflict situations as a conceptual framework for loss, no empirical studies have examined the relationships among the variables. Therefore, a co-investigator and I conducted a study of the patterns of universal conflict situations in a sample of 266 well adults. The results of that study indicate statistical support for relationships among the variables of the conflict situations at beyond the .001 level of significance. Data collection and analysis on the pattern of universal conflict situations in persons with recurrent cancer are nearly complete, and further studies to examine the pattern of these behavioral responses to loss under various conditions of change are being designed.

The need for conceptual models to guide preventive mental health services is immediate and cannot await the replication and extension of research. Mann (1972) devised a model of time-limited psychotherapy based on the construct of universal conflict patterns. I have (1982) adapted that model for working with persons with cancer, as well as with those who are experiencing other situational losses.

Universal conflict situations as a focus for primary prevention have just begun to be explored. The implications of the conceptual focus on loss as a common framework for mental health professionals is an exciting scientific, clinical, and social prospect. It demands collaboration and commitment to our shared goal of providing theory-based, cost-effective, and compassionate care in mental health. It demands a new dream.

CONCLUSION

Postulating the universality of behavioral responses to separation and loss as a conceptual focus for preventive mental health services offers a substantive approach for designing strategies that have wide applicability for primary, secondary, and tertiary levels of prevention. A caveat, however, is in order here: an explanation of the etiology of the myriad ways in which losses are perceived and their pain expressed is not implied in the framework. The impact of this limitation on the utility of the model must be addressed.

The ideal of prevention is to alter conditions in such a way that the probability of the undesired outcome is eliminated or at least significantly reduced. An underlying assumption is that there is enough information to support accurate prediction about cause and effect. Given the pervasive nondiscrete nature of the variables, demonstrating necessary and sufficient evidence of the factors that produce mental health and that eliminate mental illness is akin to unraveling the mysteries of the human condition.

The conceptual focus on loss described in universal conflict patterns does not purport to offer alternatives to the existential realities of being human; it simply states that this is the way things are. Interdisciplinary collaboration between researchers and clinicians is a prerequisite for the development of the scientific base of this conceptual framework. And since it has been noted that "therapists who have practiced for some time seem to avoid looking at other frames of reference" (Mosey 1970:226), the task of defining and refining a science of mental health may lie with those who, tempered by disillusionment in the effectiveness of established systems of theory and practice, are searching for more relevant approaches to explaining and enhancing mental health.

In acknowledging the common connection of loss as a focus for mental health services, we legitimate lonely sorrows. By designing conceptually based strategies that assist our clients — and the general public — to appreciate and integrate life's losses, we strengthen the human bond of compassion by promoting the recognition that what is most personal is, after all, universal.

The voices of the 1960s are silent. Many current solutions to social problems are simply distorted echoes of those turbulent times. And although I am no longer young or innocent enough to believe that any theory, cause, or coalition, no matter how fervent its followers, can fundamentally change the world, I still think we can make a difference.

REFERENCES

Caplan, G. 1964. *Principles of Preventive Psychiatry.* New York: Basic Books.

Fenichel, O. 1945. *Psychoanalytic Theory of Neuroses.* New York: W. W. Norton & Co.

Fitts, W. H. 1965. *Manual, Tennessee Self-Concept Scale.* Nashville: Counselor Recordings & Tests.

Gaylin, W., ed. 1968. *The Meaning of Despair.* New York: Science House.

Hartley, L. P. 1953. *The Go-Between.* London, England: Hamish Hamilton.

Klein, M. 1940. "Mourning and Its Relation to Manic-Depressive States." *International Journal of Psycho-Analysis* 21:125–153.

Mahler, M., A. Bergman, and F. Pine. 1975. *The Psychological Birth of the Human Infant.* New York: Basic Books.

Mann, J. 1973. *Time-Limited Psychotherapy.* Cambridge MA: Harvard University Press.

Mann, J. and R. Goldman. 1982. *A Casebook in Time-Limited Psychotherapy.* New York: McGraw-Hill Book Co.

Mosey, A. C. 1970. *Three Frames of Reference for Mental Health.* Thorofare NJ: Charles B. Slack.

Parens, H. 1971. *Dependence in Man.* New York: International Universities Press.

Rawnsley, M. 1982. "Brief Psychotherapy for Persons with Recurrent Cancer: A Holistic Practice Model." *Advances in Nursing Science* 69–76.

Weisman, A. D., J. W. Worden, and H. J. Sobel. 1980. "Psychosocial Screening and Intervention with Cancer Patients." *Research Report Project Omega.* Cambridge MA: Harvard University Medical School.

Winnicott, D. W. 1965. *The Maturational Processes and the Facilitating Environment.* New York: International Universities Press.

3

Emotional, Physiological, and Social Reactions to Bereavement

Tamara Ferguson

Loss of a loved one is a traumatic experience that everyone must undergo at some time. But why do some people accept their loss and carry on with their lives while others mourn for years? Lindemann (1944:141) defined bereavement as "the sudden cessation of social interaction." This definition implies that it is necessary to consider the type and quality of one's interaction with the person who died. This chapter examines research on the emotional, physiological, and social reactions of all bereaved persons and then discusses how specific problems are triggered, whether by the loss of a spouse, parent, or child.

EMOTIONAL AND PHYSIOLOGICAL REACTIONS

In his classic paper "Mourning and Melancholia," Freud (1918/1957:244–245) distinguished between mourning and melancholia, suggesting that those who are bereaved have to grieve and search for the person they have lost before they can accept the reality of their loss and proceed with living.

> Reality-testing has shown that the loved object no longer exists, and it proceeds to demand that all libido shall be withdrawn from its attachment to the object. This demand arouses understandable opposition — it is a matter of general observation that people never willingly abandon a libidinal position, not even, indeed, when a substitute is already beckoning to them. This opposition can be so intense that a turning away from reality takes place and a clinging to the object through the medium of a hallucinatory wishful psychosis. Normally, respect for reality gains the day. Nevertheless, its orders cannot be obeyed at once. They are carried out bit by bit, at great expense of time and cathetic energy and in the meantime the existence of the lost object is psychically prolonged.

Although bereaved persons are conscious of their loss, melancholic persons may not be, and their egos are impoverished. According to Waller (1966), Freud's explanation of mourning — the conflict between refusing to give up the person one loves and reality that demands that the person should be given up — is the central problem of bereavement.

Other psychoanalytic writers (Bowlby 1969, Klein 1940) proposed that the early mourning that children experience when separated from their mothers is reactivated in bereaved adults. By introjecting their loss, bereaved persons become angry at themselves; by projecting their loss, they become angry at others. Klein stated that bereaved persons once again go through the "depressed period," in which, as infants, they tried to distinguish between the "good" breast of their mothers when they were being fed and the "bad" breast when their mothers were away. Loss in adulthood reactivates these early doubts about themselves and others.

Bowlby (1963) distinguished between normal and pathological grief. In normal grief, bereaved persons go through successive periods of adjustment. In the first period, they are still striving to recover the lost object; in the second period, they experience a disorganization of their personality, accompanied by anger and despair; and in the third period, a reorganization takes place in association with the image of the lost object, as well as new objects.

Although this sequence of events does not run a smooth course, "there is plainly a discernible trend from protest through despair to some new equilibrium of feeling and behavior" (Bowlby 1963). But in pathological mourning, the bereaved cannot accept their loss, which therefore becomes repressed and unconscious and prevents them from reorganizing their lives.

At first, writers did not make a distinction between different types of loss because of the similarity of some of the grief reactions. In his study of the symptomatology and management of acute grief, Lindemann (1944) included five types of patients: psychoneurotic patients who lost a relative during the course of treatment, relatives of patients who died in the hospital, bereaved disaster victims and their close relatives, and relatives of members of the armed forces. He found that acute grief is a definite syndrome with psychological and somatic symptomatology. This syndrome may appear immediately after a crisis or it may be delayed or distorted.

Lindemann (1944) identified the following five reactions: (1) somatic distress; (2) a sense of unreality and intense preoccupation with the image of the deceased; (3) feelings of guilt; (4) hostile reactions to other people; and (5) restlessness, a loss of the "capacity to initiate and maintain organized patterns of activity." An added reaction that he observed in patients whose reactions were nearly pathological was the appearance of the traits of the deceased or of the symptoms the deceased had experienced.

Lindemann (1944:141) described the symptoms of a person experiencing acute grief:

> Common to all is the following syndrome: sensations of somatic distress occur-
> ring in waves lasting from twenty minutes to an hour at a time, a feeling of
> tightness in the throat, choking with shortness of breath, need for sighing, and
> an empty feeling in the abdomen, lack of muscular power, and an intense subjec-

tive distress described as tension or mental pain. The patient soon learns that these waves of discomfort can be precipitated by visits, by mentioning the deceased, and by receiving sympathy.

He found, further, that as soon as bereaved persons understood the grief process and were able to talk about their memories of the deceased person, their behavior improved.

Lindemann contrasted these normal reactions to bereavement with morbid reactions that he believed occur when grief is delayed or postponed or reactions are distorted. He identified eight types of distorted reactions. The first three were (1) becoming overactive without a sense of loss, (2) acquiring some of the symptoms experienced by the deceased during the last illness, and (3) developing the symptoms of a recognized medical disease:

> . . .namely, a group of psychosomatic conditions, predominantly ulcerative colitis, rheumatoid arthritis, and asthma. Extensive studies in ulcerative colitis have produced evidence that 33 out of 41 patients with ulcerative colitis developed their diseases in close time relationship to the loss of an important person. Indeed it was this observation which first gave the impetus for the present study of grief (p. 145).

The five other distorted reactions were at the level of social adjustment: (1) avoidance of social activities; (2) bitter accusations against specific persons, such as a doctor for neglect of duty; (3) hiding hostility and becoming wooden and formal; (4) inability to initiate activities or making decisions that were detrimental to the individuals' own welfare.

Lindemann made the interesting observation that patients who were prone to morbid reactions had an intense and ambivalent relationship with the deceased but could not discuss it because of loyalty or status concerns. He also noticed that patients who had anticipated their loss grieved before it occurred. His concept of "anticipatory grief" distinguishes between losses that result from chronic illnesses and are foreseen and losses that occur suddenly and unexpectedly.

Gorer (1959) asked a sample of 1,628 persons in England whether they had attended a funeral within the past five years. From this sample, he analyzed the reactions of 369 persons who had lost a parent, sibling, spouse, or child. These reactions could be categorized as different styles of mourning, such as the denial of mourning, mourning before death, unlimited mourning, and mummification (leaving everything as it was when the dead person was alive).

In the autobiographical introduction to his book, Gorer (1954) described his reactions as a child and as an adult when members of his family died. His story points to the importance of the age of the bereaved, the type and quality of the relationship with the person who has died, the circumstances of a death, the responsibilities that must be shouldered because of the loss, and cultural background in explaining some of the reactions of the bereaved.

When his father was lost on the Lusitania, Gorer was in boarding school in

England. His teachers and peers never acknowledged his loss. Indeed, he could not remember his schoolmates, the masters, or anyone else at the school speaking seriously with him about his father's death or death in general. This denial of his loss by others made Gorer prone to deny his grief. He wove fantasies in which his father had somehow escaped death and was living on a desert island somewhere in the Atlantic. Through these fantasies, he delayed acceptance of his father's death. At that time, Gorer felt as a great burden that because he was the eldest son, he had become his father's representative, and hence the caretaker of his mother and two young brothers.

Some years later, when he had become an adult, Gorer's mother died after a ravaging illness. He had anticipated her death, so that when it occurred, although he wept for her, he also felt a lessening of his responsibilities, a sense of release. Later, when his younger brother died of cancer, Gorer felt that he should have been able to prevent his death, despite the history of cancer in the family. For months afterward Gorer mourned freely and deeply.

His experiences with grief made Gorer believe that a distinction should be made between different types of death, such as the death of a father, a mother, a spouse, a sibling, or a child. Although his research indicated that the loss of a husband changes both the social and financial status of the widow, he believed that the loss of a child might cause the most devastating and enduring grief because it is contrary to the natural and expected sequence of events.

The loss of a spouse, particularly of a husband, leaves the survivor with many unfulfilled responsibilities. No longer half of a couple, the widow must determine for herself the course of her life. Furthermore, the husband was the father of her children, her social and sexual companion, and the family breadwinner — indeed, he was central to all family roles. Therefore, most surveys have focused on the loss of a husband because of the many emotional and practical problems that the widow must face.

LOSS OF A SPOUSE

It is generally believed that the first emotional reactions experienced by widows are shock, denial, anger at being abandoned, guilt that they could not prevent the death of their husbands, restlessness, sleep disturbances, and the loss of regular eating patterns, which leads, in some cases, to severe weight loss or gain. The widow finds it difficult to concentrate and make decisions. She may fear that she and her children have the same illness that caused her husband's death or be afraid of having a nervous breakdown (Ferguson 1970; Glick, Weiss, and Parks 174; Maddison and Viola 1986; Marris 1958; Parks 1972).

Health

It is common for widows to complain about their health. Marris (1958) found that 43 percent of the widows he interviewed in the East End of London thought that their health was worse than before their bereavement. Forty percent of the English widows interviewed by Hobson (1964) made the same assertion, as did two-thirds of the one hundred widows interviewed by Ferguson (1970) in the United States. Widows have been found to consult physicians more frequently (Parkes 1964a), take more medicine, and consume more alcohol than they did before their husbands died (Clayton et al 1971; Glick, Weiss, and Parkes 1974).

Maddison and Viola (1968) devised a mail questionnaire that asked widows fifty-seven questions about their health. It was answered by 132 American widows and 221 Australian widows under age sixty who had been bereaved for thirteen months, and by a control group. About 28 percent of the widows' scores showed marked deterioration of health as compared to a 4.5 percent of the control group. The widows complained not only of normal grief reactions but of dizziness, blurred vision, skin rashes, palpitations, chest pains, and frequent infections.

A study by Young, Benjamin, and Wallis (1963) found an increase of about 40 percent in the death rate among 4,486 widowers over age fifty-four during the first six months of their bereavement. In a secondary analysis of these data, Parkes, Benjamin, and Fitzgerald (1969) examined the causes of death of the widowers on the basis of their death certificates. They found that three-quarters of the increased death rate was attributable to heart disease, particularly coronary thrombosis and arteriosclerotic heart disease.

This observation of higher mortality among widows and widowers was confirmed in Reese and Lutkin's (1967) study of a semi-rural community. This survey of the close relatives of 371 residents showed that 4.8 percent died within one year after bereavement, as compared to only 0.7 percent of a comparable group of non-bereaved persons. The mortality for widows and widowers was 12 percent.

Parkes (1972:38), who extensively reviewed the physiological consequences of bereavement, concluded his analysis by saying:

> I accept the evidence that bereavement can affect physical health, and that complaints of somatic anxiety symptoms, headaches, digestive upsets, and rheumatism are likely, particularly in widows and widowers in middle ages. Finally there are certain potentially fatal conditions, such as coronary thrombosis, blood cancers, and cancer of the neck and of the womb, which seem in some cases to be precipitated or aggravated by major losses. Beyond this we cannot go. I have no doubt that further research in these areas will soon be undertaken and that many of the questions raised by these findings will be answered.

Mental Health

Several studies have found that the mental health of widows and widowers deteriorates during their bereavement. A review of the case studies of adult patients admitted to two psychiatric wards revealed that a larger-than-expected proportion of these patients had lost their spouses within six months before their admission (Parkes 1964b). The most common reaction of these patients was reactive or neurotic depression. A study by Stein and Susser (1969) indicated that a large proportion of widows and widowers were coming into psychiatric care for the first time in their lives.

Parkes (1972) compared some of the common features of grief in four studies of young and middle-aged widows (Hobson 1964; Marris 1958; Parkes 1964b; Yamamoto 1970). He found that the main difference between the psychiatric group and the other groups was that the psychiatric group had greater feelings of guilt and self-reproach. Psychiatric patients withdrew socially and found it more difficult to accept the reality of their loss than did the other bereaved spouses. Furthermore, Japanese widows whose husbands had died in car accidents had a much greater sense of the presence of the deceased than did other widows but, as Yamanoto (1970) explained, this feeling had to do with Japanese culture, which assumes the presence of ancestors.

Social Consequences

In 1979, about 12.3 million persons lost their spouses in the United States, but this figure included only 1.9 million men. Moveover, about 7.6 percent of the women aged forty-five to fifty-four were widows, but the proportion of widows aged fifty-five to sixty-four more than doubled, and it was 69.7 percent for women aged seventy-five and over (U.S. Bureau of the Census 1980: Tables 51 and 54).

There are two main reasons for the greater number of widows than of widowers: women live longer and widowers tend to remarry women who are younger than themselves. In addition, although widowhood increases with age, the number of divorces among men and women aged forty-five and over decreases, the opportunities for older widows to date and remarry are slight.

At a time when she is grieving for her husband, the widow has to make decisions about her new manner of living. If she has experienced a severe drop in income because of the loss of her husband's earning power, the widow has to decide whether to sell her house, pay her mortgage, buy life insurance, or move to another district. She may receive a great deal of advice and must evaluate carefully both the honesty and expertise of her advisers.

The financial problems of the widow who is under age sixty are different from those of the widow who is over that age. For one thing, the younger widow does not receive Social Security benefits when her children are over eighteen years (or twenty-two years if they are studying full time). The younger widow who has been a housewife for years may have to go back to work, but this is not an easy task for a woman over age forty-five who lacks special skills and experience.

The family of the widow also experiences a shift in roles. For example, the widow may start to treat her favorite son as a confidant and adviser while persisting — especially if he is young — in telling him what to do. This shift in role is confusing for the adolescent who wants to assume greater responsibility — to wear his father's mantle, as it were — and, at the same time interact with his peers.

Loneliness is another major problem for widows who are not dating. Many feel like a fifth wheel in a world of married couples, and entertaining at home or going out without an escort is difficult for the woman who depended on her husband for company.

The problems of older widows are compounded by aging. These women are concerned about their health and safety, but they may find it increasingly difficult to take care of their own needs. Lopata (1973) found that widows over age fifty-five ranked bringing up their children, particularly their sons, as their most serious problem, followed by loneliness.

Adjustment

Why do some women adjust to their problems while others become bitter, disturbed, or withdrawn from the world? Fulcomer (1942) studied the reactions of thirty-nine husbands and thirty-three wives who had lost their spouses, focusing on the first six weeks of bereavement. He found (p. 48) that the behavior of the respondents appeared to be strongly influenced by their past relationships with their spouses:

> A factor in the pre-bereavement situation which has been noted time and time again throughout the present study as an element which seems to influence the behavior of bereaved persons is the relationship previously existing between the bereaved and the deceased. This is indeed difficult to measure: determining the many phases of the relationship and then measuring their relative influences upon the responses of the bereaved person is not an easy task. But the attempt ought to be made.

Ferguson (1970) decided to test the proposition that the type of relationship that a woman had with her husband would be influential in determining her adjustment to her bereavement. Each marriage was characterized according to two criteria: (1) whether it was dominant, egalitarian, or dependent; and (2) whether the degree of conflict was high or low. The respondents were classified as dominant when they made most marital decisions and as dependent when their husband had made the decisions. Egalitarian widows had made about the same number of decisions as had their husbands. This typology was applied to five of the respondents' marital roles: financial, occupational, maternal, social, and sexual.

Ferguson (1970) found that the egalitarian widow with low marital conflict, the true "democrat," made the best adjustment. Because the dominant widow had made most of the decisions when her husband was alive, she felt that she was competent to make decisions as a widow. However, she did not realize how much her situation had changed and that before making crucial decisions she needed to decide what her new life style would be. Thus, for example, she would sell her house, buy an apartment, and then realize that her children had no room to put their toys. The dependent widow who used to turn to her husband for advice listened too much to the advice of others. For example, she might accept the offer of relatives to share their home and then realize that she had no means of transportation to go to work.

The egalitarian widow was the most prone to listen to the advice of others and then make up her own mind by taking all of her roles into consideration. Before deciding to retrain or not, she would ponder the state of her health, her age, the welfare of her children, and her social life. She did not rule out remarriage but did not pin all her hopes of a better future on her behavior in only one role, such as being a mother, having a career, or remarriage. The woman who had had a high-conflict marriage seemed to be more rigid than the woman who had had a low-conflict marriage. It was more difficult for her to tolerate the opinions of others or to trust her own opinions.

The study showed the importance of evaluating a widow's adjustment in many areas of behavior, such as religion, health, diet, education, occupation, and housing. This study and other independent studies led to the development of a rescaling theory (Ferguson et al 1981a), which was then used as a framework to give practical advice to widows in sixteen areas of behavior, or life vectors (Ferguson, Kutscher, and Kutscher 1981b).

Widowers' problems are similar to those of widows with two major differences: it is much easier for them to find female companionship than it is for widows to find male companionship. And they do not have such a severe financial problem because they can keep their jobs until retirement. They may, however, need someone to help them if their children are young.

DEATH OF A PARENT

The loss of a parent is a traumatic experience for anyone, but although it is natural to lose a parent later in life, bereavement in childhood means that the children's life patterns and their basic trust that they will not be deserted by people they love may be seriously shaken (LeShan 1976). Schowalter (1977) suggested that children under age three understand separation, but not death. After age three, preschool children believe that their parents' death stemmed from their own bad behavior. During the early school years, children begin to understand the concept of death, but it is only when they reach age ten or eleven that they fully understand the universality and permanence of death. An important distinction is whether children have lost a parent of the same or the opposite sex. If they have lost the parent of the same sex as themselves, they may take the deceased parent as a role model and try to replace that parent or may become overly attached to and dependent on the surviving parent (Ferguson 1970; Furman 1970, 1974).

Children often regress under the shock of bereavement. They frequently develop speech problems and discipline problems, and their marks in school may drop. Children experience the same grief reactions as do older people, such as shock, denial, anger, guilt, and disturbed sleep. Both LeShan (1976) and Furman (1974) stressed that it is important for children to talk about their loss so that they can realize that they are not responsible for their parents' death and have not been deserted by their deceased parents.

The long-term effects of the loss of a parent in childhood requires further study. It may be that because of a lack of confidence in the permanence of human relations, children who have lost a parent will find it more difficult later in life to establish intimate relationships with persons of the opposite sex (Hetherington 1973). These effects may depend on how well the surviving parents can adjust to their bereavement and the demands that they make on their children.

DEATH OF A CHILD

Fischoff and Brohl (1981) quoted a parent who said, "When you lose your parent, you lose your past; when you lose your child, you lose your future." But as Gorer (1959) mentioned, the more that people think of themselves primarily as mothers or fathers and only secondarily as wives or husbands, the more their self-image is desroyed. Thus, parents whose children have died have some of the same reactions as do those who have lost their spouses. Some parents and widows become bitter and believe that they will never recover from their loss, and others feel that their experience has taught them more understanding and made them recognize the kindness of others.

Marital partners may find it difficult to synchronize their moods after the loss of a child (Fischoff and Brohl 1981; Orbach 1959). They may unconsciously accuse each other of not having been able to save their child, and while one spouse becomes angry, the other one is depressed, a pattern which may ultimately lead to divorce. It seem that parents who have the most severe reaction are those who blame themselves excessively for their loss.

It would be of value to investigate whether the reactions of parents whose child died in an accident are different from those whose child died after a long terminal illness. Ferguson (1970) found that the only widows who accepted their husbands' death with equanimity were those whose husbands had died after a long, painful disease. The age of the children at death, the number and sex of the siblings, and whether the parents are young enough to have another child are all dimensions of the problem that need further investigation.

DISCUSSION

This review of the literature has shown that all bereaved persons have certain emotional and physiological reactions, such as shock, denial, anger, guilt, loneliness, disturbed sleep, restlessness, and questioning the ultimate value of life. Bereavement can also affect physical health; somatic complaints are particularly likely in middle-aged widows and widowers. In addition, certain potentially fatal conditions, such as heart disease, seem to be precipitated or aggravated by major losses. Widows and widowers may visit their doctor more frequently and take more drugs and alcohol than before their bereavement. Psychiatric symptoms may occur and require professional help.

The type and quality of the relationship between the survivor and the person who died are important in understanding the bereaved person's reactions. The widow faces many practical problems that her marriage may not have prepared her to solve. Whereas the dominant widow may rush into decisions, the dependent widow may listen too much to the advice of others. The more serene and the more egalitarian the relationship between spouses has been, the less difficult it appears to be for the survivor to come to terms with feelings of guilt and anger.

Both Ferguson (1970) and Lopata (1979) found that widows with a high level of education adjust better to their loss because they have more friends and interests. Lopata mentioned that the "multidimensional woman" experiences more social support from others. Women who put a high priority on the one role they are losing — being a wife, a daughter, or a mother — find it more difficult to accept their loss.

Silverman (1969) first realized the importance of widows being able to give advice and support to other widows. Now many self-help groups of widows exist.

The loss of a child is an excruciatingly painful experience because the parents feel that they have lost part of themselves and that their plans for the future have been destroyed. Moreover, parents may blame each other and become alienated from each other when they cannot accept the loss.

Groups and organizations for parents who have lost their children are useful. The support given by other people who are in the same situation is valuable because these people understand how important it is for the bereaved to talk about the loss as a first step toward accepting it.

Little is known about the long-term consequences of losing a parent in childhood. The age of the child, the child's understanding of what death means, and the child's recognition that he or she is not responsible for the parent's death appear to be the most important (Pincus 1974). Children need both male and female role models, and surviving parents who cling to their children may make it difficult for these children to make lives for themselves later on.

REFERENCES

Bowlby, J. 1963. "Pathological Mourning and Childhood Mourning." *Journal of the American Psychoanalytical Association* 11:500-541.

Bowlby, J. 1969. *Attachment*, vol. 1 of *Attachment and Loss*. New York: Basic Books.

Clayton, P. J., J. A. Halikas, W. L. Maurice, 1971. "The Bereavement of the Widowed." *Diseases of the Nervous System* 32:597-604.

Ferguson, T. 1970. "Conflict and the Young Widow." Unpublished Ph.D. dissertation. New York: Columbia University Press.

Ferguson, T., J. D. Ferguson, C. E. Schorer, and G. Tourney. 1981a. "Bereavement, Stress, and Rescaling Therapy." In O. S. Margolis, eds. *Acute Grief: Counseling the Bereaved*. New York: Columbia University Press, pp. 158-166.

Ferguson, T., A. H. Kutscher, and L. G. Kutscher. 1981b. "A Practical Guide for Young Widows." In *The Young Widow: Conflict and Guidelines*. New York: Arno Press.

Fischoff, J. and N. O. Brohl. 1981. *Before and After My Child Died*. Detroit MI: Emmons Fairfield.

Fulcomer, D. M. 1942. "The Adjustive Behavior of Some Recently Bereaved Spouses: A Psychosocial Study." Unpublished Ph.D. dissertation, Northwestern University.

Furman, E. 1974. *A Child's Parent Dies: Studies in Childhood Bereavement.* New Haven CT: Yale University Press.

Furman, R. A. 1970. "The Child's Reaction to Death in the Family." In B. Schoenberg, A. E. Carr, D. Peretz, and A. H. Kutscher, eds. *Loss and Grief: Psychological Management in Medical Practice.* New York: Columbia University Press, pp. 70-86.

Glick, I.O., R. S. Weiss, and G. M. Parkes. 1974. *The First Year of Bereavement.* New York: John Wiley & Sons.

Gorer, G. 1959. *Death, Grief, and Mourning in Contemporary Britain.* London, England: Cresset.

Hobson, C. J. 1964. "Widows of Blacton." *New Society* 21:517-531.

Klein, M. 1940. "Mourning and Its Relation to Manic Depressive States." *International Journal of Psycho-analysis* 21:125-153.

LeShan, E. 1976. *Learning to Say Good-Bye.* New York: Macmillan Co.

Lindemann, E. 1944. "The Symptomatology and Management of Acute Grief." *American Journal of Psychiatry* 101:141-148.

Lopata, H. Z, 1973. *Widowhood in an American City.* Cambridge MA; Schenkman Publishing Co.

Lopata, H. Z. 1979. *Women as Widows.* New York: Elsevier.

Maddison, D. and A. Viola. 1968. "The Health of Widow in the Year Following Bereavement." *Journal of Psychosomatic Research* 12:297-306.

Marris, P. 1958. *Widows and Their Families.* London, England: Routledge and Kegan Paul.

Orbach, C. E. 1959, "The Multiple Meanings of the Loss of a Child." *American Journal of Psychotherapy* 13:906-915.

Parkes, C. M. 1964a. "Effect of Bereavement on Physical and Mental Health: A Study of the Medical Records of Widows." *British Medical Journal* 2:274-279.

Parkes, C. M. 1964b. "Recent Bereavement as a Cause for Mental Illness." *British Journal of Psychiatry* 110:198-204.

Parkes, C. M. 1972. *Bereavement Studies of Grief in Adult Life.* London, England: Tavistock Publications.

Parkes, C. M., S. B. Benjamin, and R. G. Fitzgerald. 1969. "Broken Heart: A Statistical Study of Increased Mortality Among Widowers." *British Medical Journal* 1:740-746.

Pincus, L. 1974. *Death and The Family: The Importance of Mourning.* New York: Random House.

Rees, W. D., and S. G. Lutkins. 1967. "Mortality of Bereavement." *British Medical Journal* 4:13-16.

Schowalter, J. E. 1977. "Parent Death and Child Bereavement." In A. E. Carr, D. Peretz, B. Schoenberg, and A. H. Kutscher, eds. *Bereavement: Its Psychosocial Aspects.* New York: Columbia University Press, pp. 172-179.

Silverman, P. R. 1969. "The Widow-to-Widow Program: An Experiment in Preventive Intervention." *Mental Hygiene* 53:333-337.

Stein, Z. and M. W. Susser. 1969. "Widowhood and Mental Illness." *British Journal of Preventive Social Medicine* 23:106-110.

U.S. Bureau of the Census, 1980. *Statistical Abstract of the United States: 1980.* Washington D.C.: U.S. Government Printing Office.

Waller, W. 1966. "Bereavement: A Crisis of Family Dismemberment." In R. Hill, ed. The Family. New York: Holt, Rinehart & Winston, p. 476.

Yamamoto, M. D. 1970. "Culture Factors in Loneliness, Death, and Separation." *Medical Times* 98:177-183.

Young, M., B. Benjamins, and C. Wallis. 1963. "The Mortality of Widowers." *Lancet* 2:454-456.

4

Anticipatory Grief: A New Perspective

Diane Kramer

It is well understood and well documented that the death of a loved person is one of the most intensely painful experiences any human being can suffer (Bowlby 1980; Sourkes 1982; Worden 1982). Another widely held belief is that the survivor's recovery after a death depends on successful completion of the grief work (Goleman 1985; Lindemann 1944). Lindemann's (1944) seminal paper on grief stated that "normal" grief is resolved well within one year after the death. In a later study of young widows and widowers, Glick, Weiss and Parkes (1974) discovered that many subjects had not yet recovered upon reaching the one-year mark. Cox and Ford (1964) found that the risk of mortality for widows was greater during the second year of bereavement, and Joyce (1984) concluded that a survivor's way of life may be affected for as long as three years.

There is apparently no strict timetable for grieving. Moreover, a growing view of bereavement is that the complete resolution of grief may be the exception rather than the rule (DeVaul and Zisook 1976). Something goes awry, and the bereaved person is unable to do the necessary grief work. As early as 1937, Deutsch discovered that psychological wounds from a loss during childhood could fester and remain dormant for years, manifesting themselves as depressive illness during adulthood. Thus, the bereaved are a population at risk for psychological and physical illness (Bowlby 1980, Klerman and Izen 1977, Pine 1974, Worden 1982).

When early studies confirmed that the death of a family member did indeed result in serious problems, other studies began to use bereavement as a dependent variable, looking to delineate factors that affected the adjustment process. Several studies compared the effect of a spouse's sudden death with that of death that had been anticipated (Carey 1977; Clayton 1973; Ferguson 1972; Glick, Weiss and Parkes 1974). Most of this research addressed the question of whether anticipatory grief was beneficial for survivors, as if the question were, Which is better for survivors, sudden death or anticipated death? Framed this way, the question yields no answer. In widows' groups, those women whose husbands had died suddenly felt that their anguish was worse; they wished they could have had time to say good-bye. Women who had been forewarned usually felt that theirs was the worse trauma because of the helplessness and hopelessness they experienced in witnessing the suffering and gradual dying of their husbands.

Death of a spouse is rated the single greatest stress the individual faces in a lifetime (Holmes and Masuca 1970). With the reported increases in cases of cancer plus the new methods of increasing life expectancy of cancer patients, it behooves mental-health professionals to understand more about the concept of anticipatory grief.

In reviewing the literature on this subject, I found similarities as well as differences. Lindemann (1944) is universally given credit for originating the term "anticipatory grief." When Lindemann studied women whose husbands served in the armed forces during World War II, he was surprised to find that they had genuine grief reactions even though their husbands had not died. These wives were so threatened by the possibility that their husbands would die that they went through all the phases of grief and adjusted to a life without their husbands. When their husbands returned home after the war, the grief had been worked through so thoroughly that many of the women no longer loved them and wanted a divorce.

Some writers, agreeing with Lindemann's theory, defined anticipatory grief as emotional detachment from the dying person (Friedman et al 1963). Silverman (1974), who has worked extensively with widows, stated that to help a spouse grieve in advance would be inappropriate and dysfunctional. She asserted that forewarning of a death may not diminish subsequent grief.

Some writers view anticipatory grief as an adaptive mechanism (Blacher 1970, Carpenter and Hall 1974). A few take this view one step further, stating that the longer the state of dying, the greater the opportunity to accomplish in advance much, if not most, of the painful job of grieving (Glank 1974, Fulton 1972, Lehrman 1956).

Weissman (1972) noted both the benign and the harmful effects of grieving before a death occurs. He wrote about the ameliorating advantages of anticipatory grief, and admitted that there is no evidence that the bereavement after an anticipated death is more benign or short-lived than is bereavement after a sudden death. "In fact," he noted, "there is something to be said in favor of a quick, clean death. It spares survivors from the extended anguish of a death watch over the inexorable deterioration and decline of a loved one."

Most of the works cited thus far seem to be attempting to answer the question, Is anticipatory grief functional or dysfunctional? rather than to understand what goes on in the mind of the bereaved-to-be during a terminal illness. A major flaw in the literature is that anticipatory grief — a passive state — is often confused with anticipatory grief *work* — an active process. It is assumed that to be forewarned of a death is to be actively doing grief work before the death occurs. Unfortunately, few studies of anticipatory grief have been reported in the scientific literature (Kutscher, Goldberg, and Poslusny

1974). Another deficiency is that many writers operationally define anticipatory grief according to the duration of the terminal illness, but give little information about what was actually going on during the illness.

Many clinicians have compared anticipatory grief to post-death grief and have stated that their dynamics are parallel (see Fulton and Gottesman 1980) and consist of many of the same elements. Along with the similarities already recognized, I would like to suggest another. Just as conventional grief can become pathological, so can anticipatory grief, rendering the spouse of the terminally ill patient incapable of using the opportunity to do the work of grieving in advance.

Research has identified factors that are predictive of poor adjustment after the death of a spouse. Dependent, passive, and clinging personalities are indicators of a poor post-loss recovery (Freud 1917, 1957, Lopata 1970). A high degree of ambivalence, with an inability to express anger toward the dead person, are also noted as important factors (Vachon 1981, Volkan 1985). Another oft-noted variable is denial, which leads to the inability to accept the fact of death (Pine 1974, Weissman 1972). Excessive anger and guilt are two other important factors related to poor outcome. Marital relationships that are characterized by control and dominance of one member over the other are also associated with problems after the death of a spouse.

Mr. L: A Case Study

The following case example illustrates many of the foregoing points: Mr. L is a sixty-five-year-old widower, whose wife of forty years recently died of cancer. His wife had been my patient originally, and I had seen her for four sessions about two months before she died at age sixty. She was referred because she was depressed and confused about the prognosis owing to the guarded manner in which she had been given information about her condition. She was unable to swallow solid food and was often in severe pain. Her neck was quite swollen, and she felt embarrassed about her disfigurement. She spoke often of her annoyance with her husband for constantly telling her that she would be fine.

Mrs. L was an intelligent woman who had just retired from a teaching position. She was able to complain just a little about how unfair it was that she had become ill and could not do all the things she had hoped to do with her retirement. She used her therapy primarily to give herself permission to enjoy whatever time she had left, without verbalizing the fear that she might die. She felt that she could not complain to her husband because she knew he would cry if she were to admit that she was upset. I admired her courage and strength, and I liked her.

It was a struggle for Mrs. L to talk during our sessions, and the last time I saw her she had a choking spell, which frightened her. She admitted that she had been told that if she did have problems coughing or choking, it would signify that her condition had worsened. I did not see Mrs. L for a few weeks;

because it was difficult for her to speak, she had asked to be seen only once every two weeks. She did not want me to see her at home, and I honored her decision. When I did not hear from her, I called her home and was told by a housekeeper that she was in the hospital. When I called the next time, her husband told me that she had died a few days earlier.

Mr. L called me two months after Mrs. L's death, saying that he wanted to see me. He hoped that I could help him by telling him some of the things that his wife had said to me. I was not sure what he meant by that, but had some ideas that I will return to later. Mr. L had been severely depressed since his wife's death — crying, unable to sleep, losing 15 to 20 pounds because of his poor appetite. He claimed that he had no desire to live but was too much for a coward to take his own life. He said that the loneliness was killing him. He was in the habit of calling his sister, who lived 300 miles away, five or six times a day so that he could cry to her.

Mr. L felt that his problems had started with his wife's death. She had been diagnosed as having a precancerous condition more than ten years before, but he had never thought that her condition would worsen. About one year before her death, a growth had been removed and chemotherapy was administered. The growth had returned within a few months, and he and his wife were told about a type of surgery so radical that it would affect the quality of her life. The decision was made not to have this surgery, and it is not clear who made this decision. He still had no idea that her illness was life threatening; in fact, he was enraged with the doctor for daring to tell this news to them. About one month before Mrs. L died, Mr. L was told by his son that "Mother might die from this." His reaction was intense rage; he ordered his son never to say anything like that again or he would throw him out of the house.

Mr. L described his marriage of forty years as having been made in heaven. He felt that he had gone from a mother who spoiled him to a wife who continued to spoil him and cater to his every need. He believed that he and his wife had much in common and were socially inseparable. At home, he secluded himself to do his writing, and his wife protected him from the world. He recalled that he liked to be alone but only as long as his wife was within earshot so she could come when he called.

Information on Mr. L's early life disclosed that he was the first son, born after two daughters, who was catered to until his marriage. Often, during our sessions, he would say forcefully, in an angry voice, "I hate this!" "I will not tolerate this! I can't stand to be alone." He sounded like a willful two-year-old having a temper tantrum because he could not tolerate what was happening to him. He did not like to cook but did not like to eat fast foods or things that he could make for himself easily. He wanted a good home-cooked meal and could not believe that there was no one to provide it for him. Mr. L had no problem functioning at work. He was able to concentrate on his work and to relate to his colleagues. Yet the minute he returned home, he was depressed and would spend hours crying on the phone to anyone who would listen to him. His self-absorption left little room for thought about anyone else.

In the matter of his first request to me, that I share some of his wife's thoughts with him, I explored the request, hoping to find out what he needed to know. He began to get in touch with some of his guilt, suspecting that he might have been unfeeling toward her suffering. He recognized (after I suggested it) that he did not want her to die, even though she was suffering intensely. He wished that he could have kept her with him, rather than face the world alone. I think that he feared that she had complained to me about him. (She had, but of course I did not tell him.)

Looking back at the factors that are predictive of poor outcome after the death of a spouse, we can recognize several in Mr. L. A key point that alerted me to his inability to do the work of anticipatory grieving is that he could not accept the fact that his wife was dying or, later, that she had actually died. It should not come as a surprise that someone with a dependent personality would be unable to accept the fact of death. Since he did not see himself as a separate person, to acknowledge that his wife might die would be tantamount to Mr. L's facing his own death.

I have focused chiefly on personality factors within Mr. L, but one cannot look at his personality without seeing it in the context of his relationship with his wife. I do not think that Mr. L's manner of coping with Mrs. L's terminal illness and death is unique. Many couples and families cope by engaging in a similar conspiracy of silence. An extra burden was placed on Mrs. L because of her husband's verbal insistence, like an order, that she would overcome her illness.

CONCLUSION

To accept the impending death of a spouse requires the ability to adapt to change. The manner in which we adapt is formed early in life and modified by experience. It is not the purpose of this article to describe and discuss individual coping mechanisms, but to suggest that we need to know more about the coping skills of individuals and families who face the terminal illness of a family member. Thus, research is needed to identify those individuals and families who are unable to do the anticipatory grief work and, therefore, are at risk of poor adjustment after the death. Such a study would have implications for prevention because we caregivers will be able to help our patients do the effective work of anticipatory grief.

The question should not be, Is anticipatory grief functional or not functional? Rather, it should be, What are the factors that make it functional for some and dysfunctional for others? When we have that information, we can use it to help families suffering through the remissions and recurrences of their relative's illness. Remissions encourage hope, and just when the hope feels comfortable, the family is brought to despair by a recurrence. Remissions also bring closeness, and the hope that the loved one will live a while longer. New symptoms, or the recurrence of old ones, bring fears of separation and the desire to withdraw. The goal of anticipatory grief must be to help families and loved ones stay close while preparing to separate.

REFERENCES

Blacher, R. S. 1970. "Reaction to Chronic Illness." In B. Schoenberg, A. E. Carr, D. Peretz, and A. H. Kutscher. *Loss and Grief: Psychological Management in Medical Practice.* New York: Columbia University Press, 189–198.

Bowlby, J. 1980. "Loss, Sadness, and Depression," vol. 3 of *Attachment and Loss.* New York: Basic Books.

Carey, R. 1977. "The Widowed: A Year Later." *Journal of Counseling Psychology* 24(2):125–131.

Carpenter, J. and G. Hall, 1974. "Anticipatory Grief and the Disciplined Professions." In B. Schoenberg et al., eds. *Anticipatory Grief.* New York: Columbia University Press, pp. 229–236.

Clayton, P. 1973. "The Clinical Morbidity of the First Year of Bereavement: A Review." *Comprehensive Psychiatry* 14(2):151–156.

Cox, P. and J. Ford. 1964. "The Mortality of Widows Shortly After Widowhood." *Lancet* 7325 (Jan. 18):163–164.

Deutsch, H. 1937. "Absence of Grief." *Psychoanalytic Quarterly* 6(12):12–22.

DeVaul, R. and S. Zisook. 1976. "Unresolved Grief: Clinical Considerations." *Postgraduate Medicine* 59(5):267–270.

Ferguson, T. 1972. "Decision-Making and Tranquilizers in Widowhood." *Journal of Thanatology* 2:775–784.

Freud, S. 1957. "Mourning and Melancholia." In *The Complete Works of Sigmund Freud,* Vol. 14. London: Hogarth Press, pp. 237–258. (original work published in 1917).

Friedman, S. B., et. al. 1973. "Behavioral Observations of Parents Anticipating the Death of a Child." *Pediatrics* 32:610–622.

Fulton, R. and D. Gottesman. 1980. "Anticipatory Grief: A Psychosocial Concept Reconsidered." *British Journal of Psychiatry* 137:45–54.

Glick, I., R. S. Weiss, and C. M. Parkes. 1974. *The First Year of Bereavement.* New York: Wiley-Interscience.

Goleman, D. "Mourning: New Studies Affirm Its Benefit." *New York Times,* Feb. 5, 1985.

Holmes, T. H. and M. Masuda. 1970. "Life Change and Illness Susceptibility." Presented at meeting of the American Association for the Advancement of Science, Chicago (December).

Joyce, C. 1984. "A Time for Grieving." *Psychology Today* 18(Nov.):42–44.

Klerman, G. L. and J. E. Izen. 1977. "The Effects of Bereavement and Grief on Physical Health and General Well-Being." *Advances in Psychosomatic Medicine* 9:631–68.

Lehrman, S. R. 1956. "Reactions to Untimely Death." *Psychiatric Quarterly* 30:567–569.

Lindemann, E. 1944. "Symptomatology and Management of Acute Grief." *American Journal of Psychiatry* 101:141–148.

Lopata, H. 1970. "The Social Involvement of American Widows." *Behavioral Science* 14:41–47.

Pine, V. R. 1974. "Dying, Death, and Social Behavior." In B. Schoenberg et al., eds. *Anticipatory Grief.* New York: Columbia University Press, pp. 31–47.

Silverman, P. R. 1974. "Anticipatory Grief, From the Perspective of Widowhood." In B. Schoenberg et al., eds. *Anticipatory Grief.* New York: Columbia University Press, pp. 320–332.

Sourkes, B. M. 1982. *The Deepening Shade: Psychological Aspects of Life Threatening Illness.* Pittsburgh: University of Pittsburgh Press.

Vachon, M. L. S. 1981. "Type of Death as a Determinant in Acute Grief." In D. S.

Margolis et al., eds. *Acute Grief: Counseling the Bereaved.* New York: Columbia University Press, pp. 14–22.

Volkan, V. 1985. *Depressive States and Their Treatment.* Northvale NJ: Jason Aronson.

Weissman, A. D. 1973. "Coping with Untimely Death." *Psychiatry* 36:366–377.

Worden, J. W. 1982. *Grief Counseling and Grief Therapy: A Handbook for the Mental Health Practitioner.* New York: Springer Publications.

5

A Positive View of the Defense of Denial:

Implications for Treatment and Services

William Weiner

According to the traditional Freudian view, human beings are innately aggressive and need to be tamed. In this model, the psychic structures of the id, ego, and superego are involved in a power struggle. The ego represents reality and mediates between the id and the superego; the id represents the instincts of both aggression and the libidinal strivings that look for instant gratification; and the superego symbolizes internalized parental and societal values. The treatment plan for this model calls for the therapist to "make conscious what was unconscious" in the patient.

DYSFUNCTIONAL VIEW OF DENIAL

Within the Freudian perspective, denial is seen as a primitive defense the individual uses to ward off painful stimuli that produce overwhelming anxiety and thus become a threat to the individual's well-being. Despite this effect, denial is still considered to be a lower-level defense in that it negates reality. This negation is interpreted as suggesting a weak ego, which distorts reality. Thus, denial is generally seen as resistance, not as a helpful strategy for coping with a particular problem. One who is denying is seen as living in a fantasy world and is steadily encouraged to give it up in order to face the steady glare of reality.

In the literature on death and dying, one of the most important issues is that of accepting and coming to terms with one's imminent demise. To be terminally ill and think of oneself as having lived a successful life, the individual must be able to accept the idea of his or her not being. Freud, however, argued that it is impossible to imagine one's own death, since, in the unconscious, everyone is convinced of his or her own immortality. He further postulated that whenever we attempt to do so, we can perceive that we are in fact still present as spectators. Despite Freud's view, many professionals would perceive those who are not able to accept their fate as lacking in character and would feel frustrated in their consequent failure to do a significant part of their job. Thus, the task of preventive mental-health personnel is to accept the denial and to look for cracks in it. The eventual acceptance of reality, it is believed, will lead to the successful completion of the patient's life; that is, proper closure will take place.

The idea that the denial of reality is dysfunctional can be seen throughout our culture. For example, children are taught early not to daydream or make up stories that are not true, and are sometimes punished for lying and creating their own worlds. Fantasy, creative or not, is not easily tolerated in this society.

RESULTS OF CANCER STUDIES

Researchers at King's College Hospital in London evaluated the emotions of fifty-seven women after diagnosis and surgery in the early stages of breast cancer (as reported by Goldman 1985). In a follow-up study (Goldman 1985), it was found that those women who had believed that they could conquer their illness showed the best results: seven out of ten were still alive ten years later. Women who had denied their life-threatening illness, stating that they did not believe they ever had cancer, showed the next-best results: five out of ten were alive ten years later. Women who stoically accepted their disease and those who felt hopeless and helpless did the poorest. Most of these women were dead at the time of the follow-up.

It would seem that the women who took the attitude that they could overcome their life-threatening illness displayed a form of denial, and therefore that knowing and accepting the situation may not be functional for the individual. Yet many professionals, medical and otherwise, seriously question whether or not emotions can be of primary importance in the course of a serious disease. Conversely, the psychological community usually expresses the view that supportive counseling may be as important as many medical measures in treatment. Another recent study of cancer patients supported this latter view (Goldman 1985). In that study, patients who received psychotherapy along with chemotherapy had a longer life expectancy than did patients who received only chemotherapy.

Gerontologists have been stating for many years that

> The subjective feelings of an individual are often better indices of how the individual will function than a physical examination. It is as though when people become old they accommodate to physical disease and discomfort. The old person who feels he is functioning well, irrespective of clinical pathology, tends on the whole to behave as if he were well (Sheldon, McEwan, and Ryser 1975:106).

Palmore's (1982) study found that the strongest predictor of longevity for men was self-rating of their health; for women, the strongest predictor was degree of satisfaction with their health. This study pointed out that the older person who is able to compensate and to minimize impairments has a longer life expectancy. It seems that the subjective, hopeful feelings of the elderly are more fruitful predictors than is external reality.

In light of these and other research findings, why does the denial of reality have such a negative connotation in the mental-health community and in this culture? Philosophers and scientists have long debated the nature of reality and pondered, but not resolved, the question of whether an event that is not perceived by an observer is indeed "real."

The notion that reality is fragile and anxiety-producing occurred to Weisman (1972), who went to the core of the problem in stating that when individuals deny a serious illness, they are in effect refuting the reality of the observer. This may be one reason why mental-health professionals who work with terminally ill patients may feel that it is urgent for patients to come to terms with and accept their life-threatening illness.

The positive research findings on the use of denial, on the one hand, and the need of the observer to break through the defense of denial, on the other hand, seem to call for a re-evaluation of the "primitiveness" of denial as well as of treatment techniques.

THE VIEW OF KOHUT

In an attempt to explore the issue of denial, I will, in the remainder of this chapter, present Kohut's (1971) view of humanity. This discussion includes a reinterpretation of pathology, which links Kohut's interpretation to implications for professionals who offer preventive mental health services.

Kohut's self-psychology replaces the psychic structures of the ego, id, and superego with the concept of the nuclear self with which the child is born. In this view, people have no innate aggressive drives; their aggressive acts are responses to an unresponsive environment. From early on, the child's sense of self develops through experiences with self-objects. (A self-object, according to this view, is an object outside the self that is experienced as part of the self.) The earliest self-objects are parental figures on whom the child is dependent. The child's self will develop cohesively if, through the parental figures, it is properly nourished.

Kohut (1971) also developed the idea of a bipolar self. In this view, the child is usually first mirrored by the mother; this mirroring allows the child's healthy grandiosity to flourish. The male parental figure, usually the second part of this bipolar self, permits the child to idealize him — to see him as a strong but benign and available object. If the child does not receive adequate mirroring or is not allowed to idealize the parental figure, the child's self becomes fragmented, which causes low self-esteem and narcissistic rage. The fragmented self responds to the slightest provocation, real or not, with aggression — an act that reflects the internal disintegration the child is experiencing.

The treatment plan in this model is different from that in the traditional Freudian view. A cohesive self is reconstructed and strengthened by corrective emotional experiences in which the therapist makes up for the nonresponsiveness experienced by the patient in earlier life. The therapist achieves this by mirroring the individual and allowing for idealization to take place. The most crucial role of the therapist in self psychology is to understand and be supportive of the patient's wishes, needs, and experiences.

Self psychology believes that whatever the person does should be seen as necessary at that time; this is, the therapist must understand and empathize with the patient's subjective interpretation of reality. For example, a terminally ill patient may come to the point of expressing a wish to die. The therapist might respond by expressing understanding of the patient's feelings under the circumstances, and by stating that if the therapist were to have all these problems, he or she might not do as well as the patient is doing. The goal of the mirroring is to heighten the person's self-esteem. Even if a person denies the seriousness of an illness and talks about some unrealistic plans for the future, the therapist still empathizes with the patient's wishes for the future, explores those wishes with the patient, and allows the patient to expand on them.

Kohut's concept of understanding the other person's subjective world would, of necessity, exclude the notion of making conscious what is unconscious. In other words, the therapist always stays where the patient is in the situation. One implication of this idea is that denial may be a necessary coping device for the critically ill and may be useful in everyday living.

Weisman (1972) stated that anyone whose survival and self-esteem are threatened is likely to use denial. Further, he made many references to loss of self-esteem among those who are dying. To me, the concept of self appears to be synonymous with self-esteem. It seems to follow, then, that the self-esteem would need to be preserved at all costs. This appears to be essential not only for mental health but also for the prolongation of life itself.

CONCLUSION

If it is true that denial is an effective coping device in many situations, we professionals may need to examine and re-evaluate our treatment approach. Obviously, further research studies should be attempted to test the validity of this hypothesis. In practice, the therapist can use this approach even with a single client and test the changes it could possibly bring about.

For this treatment plan to be most effective, our culture at large would also have to begin looking at denial in a different, more positive, light. As pointed out earlier, from infancy on, we are indoctrinated with the idea that denial is pathological. We come to believe that salvation can come about only by facing the "truth" that is imposed and interpreted by others, while squelching our own. It may be that stressing the full value of the individual and the individual's own acceptance of the world may lead to positive and unexpected changes throughout the person's lifespan.

REFERENCES

Goldman, D. 1985. "Strong Emotional Responses to Disease May Bolster Patient's Immune System." *New York Times*, Section C1, October 22.

Kohut, H. 1971. *The Analysis of the Self.* New York: International Universities Press.

Palmore, E.B. 1982. "Predictions of the Longevity Difference: A 25-Year Follow-Up." *The Gerontologist* 22(6):733-742.

Sheldon, A., McEwan, P.J.M. and Ryser, C.P. 1975. *Retirement Patterns and Predictions.* Washington DC: U.S. Department of Health, Education, and Welfare.

Weisman, A.D. 1972. *Dying and Denying: A Psychiatric Study of Terminality.* New York: Behavioral Publications.

ADDITIONAL READING

Fenichel, O. 1945. *The Psychoanalytic Theory of Neurosis.* New York: W.W. Norton & Co.

Killilea, A.G. 1985. "Nuclearism and the Denial of Death." *Death Studies* 9(3–4):254–263.

Lichtenberg, J.D. and Kaplan, S. eds. 1983. *Reflections on Self Psychology.* Hillsdale NJ: Analytic Press.

Stepansky, P.E. and A. Goldberg, eds. 1984 *Kohut's Legacy.* Hillsdale NJ: Analytic Press.

White, M.T. and M.B. Weiner. 1986. *The Theory and Practice of Self Psychology.* New York: Brunner/Mazel.

6

Family Coping With Stressors:

A Theoretical Approach

William J. Sobotor

Only within recent years has interest in illness as a specific aspect of family stress been generated in the literature. This chapter relies, therefore, not only on the literature related to illness-specific stressors but also on concepts of the family and on other stressors. It discusses how these other factors can be adapted to fit the illness-as-stressor model.

CONCEPTS OF THE FAMILY

Family theorists and researchers have identified specific characteristics of the family that are important for this discussion. These concepts include the interdependence of family members, the family's selective maintenance of boundaries, the family's ability to modify its structure in reaction to change, and the family as a task-performance group.

Interdependence of family members implies not only a complementarity of roles but the development of specific subsystems within the family group. Such subsystems include the marital dyad, relationships among siblings, and parent–child relationships. Understanding that the family is indeed selective in its maintenance of boundaries has been reinforced by the work of Boss (1980), which pointed to a more flexible type of boundary maintained by the family. The family's adaptability to change and modification is perhaps one of the reasons for its continued survival as an institution. It is important to remember that not only will the family change in reaction to external pressures or events, but that the family is capable of initiating change.

The family as a task-performance group is an especially important concept in developmental theory. Among the tasks generally assigned to the family by family scholars are (1) the physical maintenance of family members, (2) the socialization of family members for roles in the family and other groups, (3) the maintenance of family members' motivation to perform familial and other roles, (4) the maintenance of social control both within the family and between family members and outsiders, and (5) the addition of family members through reproduction or adoption and the release of those members, when they are mature, into society. The family's performance is especially important when one looks at the family as it moves through the family life cycle.

As Feldman and Feldman (1975) pointed out, the word "cycle" refers to a repeated sequence of events. A family's existence over time does not actually constitute a cycle, since that would imply that the same group of people continuously and successively experiences the same types of events. In reality, a family starts with the marital dyad and progresses through successive stages until the death of the initial spouses. For this reason, the term "family life career" will be used instead of "family life cycle."

Stages of the Family Life Career

Intricately linked to the family career is the concept of stage, which allows one to analyze similar families who occupy similar positions in the family career. A stage is a mere division in the life or existence of the family which has distinctive characteristics that enable us to separate it from other stages.

One of the more popular staging systems for the family life career is that of Duvall (1971). This system is based on the following criteria: the changes in the number of members in the family, the developmental stages of the oldest child, and the retirement status of the husband-father. This staging system includes (1) beginning families (married couples without children), (2) childbearing families (in which the oldest child is less than thirty months old), (3) families with preschool children (in which the oldest child is under six yeas of age), (4) families with school-age children (in which the oldest child is six to thirteen years old), (5) families with teenagers (in which the oldest child is thirteen to twenty years), (6) families as launching centers (in which the first child has left home and the last child is leaving home), (7) families in the middle years (from empty nest to retirement), and (8) aging familes (from retirement to the death of both spouses).

This staging system has come under some discussion. Glick (1977) argued that because about 4 percent of the married women born between 1940 and 1950 will not have children, they will have no stages in their family life career that involve children. At the same time, our society is faced with the complexity of increased divorce rates, increased rates of remarriage, and, therefore, an increase in the number of blended families. Such families have unique characteristics that are based on the family members' separate experiences in their families of origin, in their first marriages, and in the blended family. For all practical purposes, however, I will consider the norm to be Duvall's criteria and her resultant stages.

Caution must be exercised, however, in using these criteria, since changes in the median ages of people at various stages of the life career have become evident. For example, many women are delaying the birth of their first child and are shortening the span of their childbearing years. In addition, the increase in the median length of successful marriages, coupled with the reduced child-rearing period, will result in a longer empty-nest period and will allow many couples to spend more time together after their last child has left home.

Developmental Tasks

Specific developmental tasks involved in each stage of the family life career are another important consideration.

In **Stage 1,** the beginning family's primary tasks include forming a new unit, developing solidarity as a couple, and negotiating the various marital roles that must be filled.

In **Stage 2,** families who are experiencing the birth of children find that although parenting may provide satisfaction and rewards, some of the previous marital roles must take second place. For example, the wife-mother must now devote more time to the care of the infant and often is employed outside the home. The husband-father may also participate in child care and has external job and societal pressures to deal with. The original dyad must now incorporate additional members; the result is changes in roles and new responsibilities.

In **Stage 3,** families with preschool children must provide for the socialization of these children as well as continue to satisfy the children's basic needs. The emerging personalities of the children must be accepted into the family system.

In **Stage 4,** families with school-age children must provide adequate educational opportunities for their children and become involved in such education-related activities as the PTA, Little League, and so forth. Such seemingly innocuous activities demand more of their time and a further expansion of the parental role. Parents must also encourage their children's involvement with school, friends, sports, other recreational activities and the like, and incorporate feedback from those sources.

In **Stage 5,** families with teenagers must begin to accept the growing independence of their children and prepare for the children's eventual leave-taking. Many authorities argue that this is the most painful stage of parenting because the increasingly independent desires of the teenagers come into conflict with the parents' methods of childrearing and their attempts to continue the children's dependence on them. Teenagers are of course dealing with the physical and emotional changes that occur during puberty.

In **Stage 6,** the family as a launching center must not only permit the children to become independent and leave the family home, but must prepare to incorporate their children's marital partners and eventual grandchildren.

In **Stage 7,** families in the middle years continue to incorporate new members in the form of grandchildren and in-laws and experience the loss of other family members through death. The original dyad must continue to redefine the relationship. This re-evaluation is necessary, since, after many years of their roles and responsibilities as wife-mother and husband-father, they now have returned to their wife–husband roles.

In **Stage 9,** the main developmental task of aging families is to accept retirement, with its diminished income; to deal with the couple's possible decline in physical status; and to prepare for the eventual death of one of the spouses. Many times, the aging couple must also accept increased dependence on their children because of their physical decline. The older couple has also experienced and must resolve the loss of parents, siblings, and friends.

Gartner, Fulmer, Weinshal, and Goldklank (1978) reported the effects of developmental or transitional events on the mental health of family members. For example, they observed that if the presenting patient was a spouse in an intact marriage, the patient most often would be a woman in her early thirties and suffering from depression. Gartner and colleagues stated that such depression was a result of the culturally defined crisis surrounding a female's thirtieth birthday combined with the fact that these women's children had all begun school. They concluded that the transitional issues of sending children to school (with reduced demands on the caretaker) and the "end of youth" provoked the crisis.

For another example, they found that the typical patient who was a child of an intact couple was usually a male in his mid-twenties, with chronic schizophrenia that dated back to late childhood or adolescence. One explanation for this finding was that these youths' emotional dependence on their parents prevented them from adequately preparing for a career, education, and independence.

Furthermore, they found that if the patient was a child of a single parent, it was likely that the child would be female, under age thirty, and suffering from a chronic or reactive disorder that began during adolescence. The inability to achieve adequate independence from the single parent was seen as the critical factor.

Single adults who were patients were generally females over the age of thirty whose symptoms had first appeared at or around age thirty. Critical factors that caused their symptoms included the death of a parent or spouse, or divorce. These examples from the work of Gartner and colleagues (1978) make clear the importance of accomplishing the appropriate developmental tasks. One can only speculate about how these subjects would have fared had there been a history of a long, debilitating illness in their families in addition to the normative events they experienced.

IMPACT OF ILLNESS

The impact of illness on the family system cannot easily be analyzed. Part of the difficulty rests in the time of the illness and the position of the family in its life career. If one uses Hill's classical conceptualization of a crisis event, with A (the event) interacting with B (the family's crisis-meeting resources) interacting with C (the family's definition of the event) producing X (the crisis), one can appreciate how the family's crisis-meeting resources and the definition of the event will be directly dependent on the family's position in the family life career (see Figure 1).

FIGURE 1
Schematic representation of Hill's model.

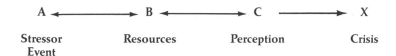

These factors are compounded by the fact that no crisis occurs in isolation. Carter and McGoldrick (1980) provided a clear schematic illustration of the compound effect of stressors on the family system. They stated that families are exposed to both vertical and horizontal stressors. Vertical stressors include the family's attitudes, taboos, expectations, and developmental issues. Horizontal stressors include the anxieties and stress produced by changes that occur in the family as it moves through time, coping with these changes, and the resultant transitions in the family life career. Horizontal stressors include both predictable developmental stressors for normative events as well as unpredictable events, including death, the birth of defective children, chronic illness, war, and so forth. According to Carter and McGoldrick's framework, the family is a group of people who move through time and occupy a point that is at an intersection between horizontal and vertical stressors.

Terkelsen (1980) further defined horizontal stressors as normative and paranormative events. Included in the normative category are marriage; the birth of children; children's entrance into school, adolescence, or adulthood; the birth of grandchildren; and retirement. In the paranormative category are events that tend to modify the normative functions of the family. They include miscarriage, separation and divorce, illness, disability and death, the relocation of the household, and changes in socioeconomic status. Normative events happen to most families and are derived directly from procreative and child-rearing functions. Paranormative events occur frequently but not universally. The difficulty is that when a paranormative event occurs, it must be dealt with in addition to the normative events.

In looking at illness as a paranormative event, one sees that the disruption of the family system is affected by a number of factors, such as the timing of the illness in the family life course, the nature of the illness, the openness and communication patterns in the family system, and the role position of the ill member.

Coupled with these factors is the concept of limited linkage, introduced by Magrabi and Marshall (1965). This concept implies that as the family moves through time, the action it takes to resolve or ignore issues at a given point will subsequently limit the alternatives available for resolving additional problems later. When chronic illness impinges on the family and hinders the attainment of the family's developmental goals, the effects of the family's action or inaction will continue to be felt as the family moves through additional developmental tasks in different stages of the life career.

Another concept to be considered when investigating the impact of chronic illness on the family is that of Glaser and Strauss (1968), who described the course of events related to an illness as an individual's and family's passage through time. Glaser and Strauss labeled this course of events the trajectory of the illness and demonstrated that this trajectory or path is not smooth or even. On the contrary, the emotional impact of the situation can resemble a ride on a roller coaster. As the family moves from the point of the diagnosis through the course of the illness, with recurrence or continued intensification of the symptoms, the roller-coaster effect is demonstrated even more. Subsequent events in the illness leave the family functioning at a less-than-optimal emotional level.

THE CRISIS OF CHRONIC ILLNESS

The impact of chronic illness upon a family depends in part on how the family perceives the crisis. When the illness is first diagnosed, the crisis is perceived differently from, say, a separation crisis. It is more blurred, since it depends, to a great extent, on communication patterns within the family and the level of understanding of family members. As time passes, boundaries between subsystems will begin to fluctuate. If the patient is a parent, for example, the family becomes more dependent on the children because the sick parent is unable to fulfill some obligations of the parental role. Thus, children will have to display increased independence and may be forced to assume some of the duties and responsibilities of the parental role. At this point, secondary crises may occur in the family system.

The family members are required to define the illness. Will they perceive the chronically ill parent to be sick or not sick? Perceptions of the patient as not sick are possible with certain diagnoses. For example, many dialysis patients can lead normal lives except when required to go for their treatments. Thus, family members and others may perceive them as not being sick, despite the presence of life-threatening chronic illness. Depending on the way family members define or label the diagnosed individual, different outcomes (reorganizations) will ensue. If the family decides the event is life-threatening, certain reorganizations will take place. If, despite medical advice, the family refuses to accept the diagnosis and chooses to pretend that the illness is less than life threatening, other patterns will emerge that will later have adverse effects upon the family system. This is an example of the concept of limited linkage in practice.

Data of the U.S. Bureau of Vital Statistics show that diseases of degeneration have replaced diseases of contagion as the leading cause of death. Heart disease, malignant neoplasms, and cerebral vascular disease are among the leading causes of death in people aged twenty-five and over. A clear implication is that in many families, at least one member will be ill for a long time. The cumulative effect of the stresses this creates within the family system is bound to be felt at some point.

Similarly, a diagnosis will have different ramifications, depending on the family's position in its life career. For example, cerebral vascular disease will have different consequences for a seventy-year-old than for a forty-five-year-old person. In the former situation, cerebral vascular disease is not unusual. The person, in all likelihood, would have been retired and his or her children established in their own households. Someone with the same diagnosis at age forty-five would still be gainfully employed and might well be the family breadwinner. Furthermore, because many couples now have children later in life, children may still be residing in the parental household. In such a case, the effects would be multiplied and intervention techniques would have to take this into account.

COPING WITH CHRONICALLY ILL CHILDREN

In children aged one to four years, congenital anomalies and malignant neoplasms are sometimes listed as the leading causes of death, but the major cause of death in this age group is accidents. One can appreciate the difference in the stress placed on the family when a child dies from an accident or from a malignant neoplasm. In accidental death, the initial shock and trauma are overwhelming, but it is an immediate crisis, and the family will begin its reorganization pattern. With a malignant neoplasm, however, the family must endure a period of continued stress that could alter its developmental course. In this situation, both the parents and the other children could experience many of the negative consequences of a chronic illness prior to the ill child's death.

Patterson (1985) analyzed the factors associated with a family's ability to comply with home care for children with cystic fibrosis. She found that the age of the patient had an inverse effect on compliance. Families with female patients showed greater compliance, as well as a pattern of decreased outside recreational activities. If the mother was not employed outside the home and if both parents were involved in home care, there was increased compliance. In "expressive" families, in which open communication was encouraged, greater compliance was manifest. Of major note is her finding that families who defined the illness as manageable were more compliant. Patterson attributed parents' greater compliance with the care of older children primarily to the build-up of stresses as well as to the progression of the disease with time. It could be that families in which older children were ill were facing issues far different from those faced by families at less advanced stages of the illness.

McCubbin and colleagues (1983) found three distinct parental coping patterns in caring for a chronically ill child: (1) maintaining family integration and cooperation with an optimistic definition of the situation; (2) maintaining social support, self-esteem, and psychological stability; and (3) understanding the medical situation through communication with other parents and consultation with the medical staff. In further analyses of the data, McCubbin and colleagues found distinct differences between mothers' and fathers' coping mechanisms. For example, the mother's effort to maintain integration, cooperation, and optimism was directly related to improvements in the child's health. For the father, improvement in the child's health tended to affect efforts to maintain social support, self-esteem, and psychological stability. In addition, the higher the family income, the greater was the father's involvement in the medical aspects of child care and the greater the mother's efforts to gain support and to maintain self-esteem.

As a result of their study, McCubbin and colleagues (1983) suggested that parental coping should be a legitimate concern of health educators, physicians, nurses, and allied health professionals. Since the coping of the mother and father seem complementary, the authors thought that some families may be at a greater risk than others. For example, in single-parent families there is no spouse to share the responsibility of coping with the situation. The child's age is also important: with the child's increasing age, there was a negative relationship with the mother's effort to maintain social support and a positive relationship with the father's efforts to understand medical issues. Families with low income are also at increased risk.

Barbarin, Hughes, and Chester (1985) investigated stress and coping among parents of children with cancer. Their respondents (32 married couples) reported that the family's cohesion was apparently strengthened by their experience and that spouses were the most important source of support. These authors cautioned, however, that as the number of hospitalizations increased, the perception of support from the spouse and the quality of the marrige decreased. The wife's perception of support from her husband was directly related to his involvement in the care of the child; the husband's perception of support from his wife was related to her being at home rather than at the hospital.

In the study by Barbarin, Hughes, and Chester (1985), most respondents indicated that the quality of their marriages or family life had improved after the child's illness was diagnosed. Only 5 percent of the respondents reported less positive feelings toward their spouse than before their child's diagnosis. In addition, the wives' and husbands' ratings of marital quality and support from their spouse agreed closely with each other. Analyzing the effect of their spouse's involvement in medical care, most of the respondents indicated that the wife had primary responsibility for monitoring the child's care. The data also indicated that the husband's involvement in the child's care was not related to the wife's perception of her husband's support. However, the time wives spent with the child in the hospital was negatively associated with the husbands' perceptions of their wives' support but not with the quality of the marriage. This finding is interesting, since of the sixty respondents who were interviewed, about twenty indicated that their family life had become generally better, and twelve reported that their marriages had improved. These respondents were evidently able to see a positive growth from the family crisis.

It would be interesting to do a follow-up study with this same sample because of the pattern of diagnoses among the children. The vast majority of youngsters in the study had non-controllable types of cancer. Thirty-three percent had leukemias; 18 percent had cancers of the brain and central nervous system; and 12.5 percent had bone tumors. The minority of children were diagnosed as having either lymphomas or Wilms' tumors, which would have more favorable prognoses. It may well be, as the authors suggested, that the findings would have been different if the study had included a number of parents whose children had died. Because the parents were focusing on the children's survival, they may have put other stressors in the background. It would be interesting in a follow-up study to see if the McCubbin and Patterson (1984) pile-up effect would surface.

EFFECTS OF GENDER AND PERCEPTION OF BURDEN

Barbarin, Hughes and Chester (1985) also discussed some gender-related findings. For the wives, spousal support was associated with the husbands' participation in the care of the ill children, which, as they pointed out, is traditionally defined as a mother's responsibility. The wives' perceptions of the quality of their marriages were also related to the husbands' active involvement in the children's medical care and to the husbands' obtaining information about the illness and its treatment. In this sample, however, it was the wives who reported assuming almost sole responsibility for staying with their children in the hospital. The husbands reported that they felt that the quality of their marriages was diminished if their wives had to spend excessive time at the hospital. The more frequently the wives were staying with the children in the hospital, the less support the husbands perceived. The authors concluded that for both wives and husbands the evaluation of marital functioning was associated with circumstances that would free the mother from having to spend significant amounts of time away from home.

Patterson and McCubbin (1984) investigated the effect of gender role on the ability to cope. Although their study was concerned with the effect of long-term separation of spouses because of military duty, the results can be applied to other areas of coping among spouses. Patterson and McCubbin found that those wives who described themselves as being androgynous in their gender-role orientation experienced minimal distress from their husbands' extended absence. Wives who reported a lower level of distress used a balanced coping strategy in which they used many coping patterns and were thus able to address the needs of the family system, with attention to personal growth and individual emotional needs.

In analyzing their results, Patterson and McCubbin found that by applying the AA-BB-CC-XX model of family behavior (McCubbin and Olson 1984), they were able to view coping as the interaction of resources and family perceptions, whereby non-primary caregivers and family members in the community were used to meet the pile-up of demands that resulted from the crisis. The results of this study tie in nicely with those of the study by Barbarin, Hughes, and Chester (1985), wherein the quality of the marriage seemed to be inversely related to the wives' performance of traditional maternal roles. It may well be that people would cope better if they had an androgynous outlook on roles. Such an outlook would minimize role confusion and the disorganization that occurs in the family system during a stressful event because roles that are no longer being fulfilled by a family member of a particular sex could be picked up by another family member of the opposite sex.

Pratt and colleagues (1985) studied the effect of caring for patients with Alzheimer's disease. Two groups of caregivers were studied — those who used support groups and those who did not. The final sample had 240 caregivers; 61 percent participated in support groups and 39 percent did not. Forty-four percent were caregivers to husbands (with a mean age of 72.9 years); 14 percent were caregivers to wives (with a mean age of 72.6 years); 30 percent were caregivers to parents (the mean age of the mothers was 77.5 years and that of the fathers was 76.7 years); and 12 percent were caregivers to other relatives (in-laws, siblings, and aunts). Sixty-one percent of the patients were not institutionalized.

Among the significant findings was the relationship between the perceived burden and the caregiver's health status. The better the caregivers perceived their health to be, the less burden they felt. Confidence in problem solving and reframing were significantly related to the scores on perceptions of the burden being carried. Significant external coping strategies included spiritual and kin-network support. The definition of the illness by the caregivers as well as their sense of family support seem to be critical in minimizing the perceived burden.

TWO MODELS OF COPING

The AA-BB-CC-XX model (of McCubbin and Olson 1984) was presented as an expanded version of Hill's original crisis model. This expanded model includes AA, the family's pile-up of life events and stressors over time; BB, the family's strengthening or building of resources within the family and in transactions with the community; CC, the family's perception of the stressor and related changes in the family; and XX, the end state of family adaptation or breakdown following a crisis (see Figure 2).

Another concept for understanding the differential impact of illness on the family system is that provided by Bain (1978). Bain argued that a family's capacity to cope with a transition or change is inversely proportional to the transitional density (TD) and the magnitude of role changes (RC) involved in the particular transition or change, and is directly proportional to the degree of organization in the formal social container (FSC) within which the transition or change occurs and the size and relevance of the family's social network (SN). Bain defined transitional density as the sum total of changes and transitions

FIGURE 2
Schematic representation of McCubbin and Olson's model.

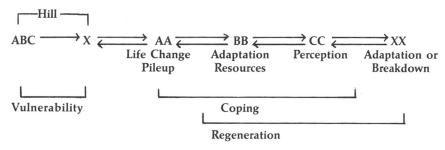

that have occurred in the family within a given time. The magnitude of the role changes is defined as shift in role structure caused by the particular transition or change that must take place within the family system. The formal social container is defined as that organization, such as a hospital, school, or self-help group, within which the change took place or with which the family had contact because of the change. The family's social network is defined as the sum total of supports that are available to the family in the form of relatives, friends, neighbors, co-workers, and other colleagues. Bain's model can be expressed as follows:

$$FC = \frac{FSC.SN}{TD.RC}$$

It is important to note that as the family moves through its life career, its social network will change because of the cumulative effect of normal transitions the family has made. With time, the family will add new acquaintances, friends, work places, and so forth. Through marriages, in-laws will be added to the family, whereas other relatives will be removed through divorce or death. One can appreciate, then, that the social network is a dynamic group that changes as the family changes.

Space precludes a lengthy discussion of each stage of the family life career. The following conclusions are offered as generalities that may be applied to any family throughout the course of life. Thus, the impact of a chronic illness on the family system will vary as a result of the following factors:

- *The type of illness and the natural course of events of that illness.* With cancer, for example, there is considerable uncertainty. Cancer involves lengthy treatment and the outcome may remain in doubt. In cardiovascular disease, recent technological advances could affect the outcome; these advances could also result in additional stresses and, possibly, additional crises.
- *The stage of the illness at the time of diagnosis.* Knowledge of it would give the family some idea of the expected course of events and would give

the medical community some idea of the severity of the illness and its prognosis.

- *The makeup of the family system.* For example, if the family is the original marital dyad, the impact will be different than if the family includes the parents and three or four children. As the illness affects one family member, it will affect the interactions among all. These interactions will in turn cause reactions that reverberate throughout the family system. Furthermore, if the family has an extended kin network that is available for emotional and physical support, the outcome would be different than if the family is isolated by geography or other factors.

- *The particular role occupied by the person who is ill.* If this person is the husband–father and he provides the main financial support for the family, the ramifications of a chronic debilitating illness for him will be much different than if the wife–mother, who may not have been employed outside the home, were the patient. If the father were ill, the mother would have to assume many of the external roles that the father formerly occupied, including outside employment, while maintaining her role responsibilities. If the mother were ill, then the father, in addition to his outside employment and responsibilities, would have to take on many of the traditionally maternal or nurturing functions of the mother's role. Such changes in roles are dependent on the availability, willingness, and ability of other family members to assume the roles of the ill member. If other members are not able to do so, the family will experience additional stressors.

- *The point in the individual's life span at which the illness occurs.* If the illness is considered to be at variance with the normal course of events, it will have different consequences than if it was to be expected because of the person's chronological age. The impact of cancer on a young mother with children at home is clearly different from the impact of cancer on an elderly grandmother because of the different roles and responsibilities of the two women.

Imig's (1981) investigation of accumulated stresses and interpersonal effectiveness in the family found that husbands' and wives' interpretations of the impact of life changes vary. Imig found some slight evidence that husbands but not wives experience a sense of loss of control. Such differences in the perceptions of events may lead to an inappropriate fulfillment of role responsibilities by one of the marital partners.

A MODEL OF THE FAMILY HEALTH CYCLE

Doherty and McCubbin (1985) presented a concise model of family health and illness. The model includes the following phases: (1) the promotion of health and the reduction of risks in the family, (2) the family's vulnerability and the onset of the illness, (3) the family's appraisal of the illness, (4) the family's acute response, (5) the family and the health care system, and (6) the family's adaptation to the illness.

Phase 1 comprises the identification and shaping of environmental, social, psychological, and personal factors within or surrounding the family that are thought to promote wellness. Phase 2 encompasses those life events or experiences that may precipitate an episode of an illness. Phase 3 involves the family's efforts to give definition and meaning to the actual illness. Phase 4 incorporates the immediate emotional and interactional aftermath for the family once the illness experience has been felt. Phase 5 refers to the family's decision whether to seek outside help for the illness or to handle it within the family. Phase 6 refers to the long-term impact of illness on the family and to the role of the family in the rehabilitation and recovery of the ill member.

CONCLUSION

The effects of chronic illness on the family system are better understood if we return to the McCubbin-Olson (1984) and Bain (1978) models. Only through a synthesis of the two will we come closer to predicting the outcome for families who experience normative and concurrent paranormative events. The life changes and pile-up effect (AA) of the McCubbin and Olson model are comparable to transitional density (TD) and role change (RC) of the Bain model. Adaptation and resources (BB) are similar to the formal social container (FSC) and social network (SN). Through substitution, one arrives at a workable, predictive formula (see Figure 3).

FIGURE 3
Synthesis of McCubbin-Olson and Bain models.

(TD.RC)   (FSC.SN)   (FC)   (XX)   (BB)

$$A A \rightleftharpoons BB \rightleftharpoons CC \rightleftharpoons X X \qquad FC \quad = \quad \dfrac{FSC.SN}{TD.RC}$$
$$(AA)$$

Therefore, $\dfrac{BB.CC}{AA} = XX$

The synthesized model accounts not only for the historical background of the family system but for the changes in the family system and in the network interacting with the family. The stage in the family life career is addressed by the function BB/AA. Since the model is dynamic, it will account for all normative and paranormative changes the family experiences.

Doherty (1985) called for more descriptive and developmental involvement of the social sciences in health care. Perhaps this new synthesis can serve to advance such an endeavor.

REFERENCES

Bain, A. 1978. "The Capacities of Families to Cope with Transition: A Theoretical Essay." *Human Relations* 31:675–688.

Barbarin, O., D. Hughes, and M. Chester. 1985. "Stress, Coping, and Marital Coping Among Parents of Children with Cancer." *Journal of Marriage and the Family* 47:474–480.

Boss, P. 1980. "Normative Family Stress: Family Boundary Changes Across the Life Span." *Family Relations* 219:445–480.

Carter, E. and M. McGoldrick. 1980. "The Family Life Cycle and Family Therapy: An Overview." In E. Carter and M. McGoldrick, eds. *The Family Life Cycle: A Framework for Family Therapy*. New York: Gardner Press, pp. 3–20.

Duvall, E.M. 1971. *Family Development*. Philadelphia PA: J. B. Lippincott, pp. 106–107.

Doherty, W. 1985. "Family Interaction in Health Care." *Family Relations* 34:129–137.

Doherty, W. and H. McCubbin, 1985. "Families and Health Care: An Emerging Arena of Theory, Research and Clinical Interaction." *Family Relations* 34:5–11.

Feldman, H. and M. Feldman. 1975. "The Family Life Cycle: Some Suggestions for Recycling." *Journal of Marriage and the Family* 37:277–283.

Gartner, R., R. Fulmer, M. Weinshal, and S. Goldklank. 1978. "The Family Life Cycle: Developmental Crises and Their Structural Impact on Families in a Community Mental Health Center." *Family Process* 17:47–58.

Glaser, B. and A. Strauss. 1968. *A Time for Dying*. Chicago: Aldine Press.

Glick, P. 1977. "Updating the Life Cycle of the Family." *Journal of Marriage and the Family* 39:5–13.

Imig, D. 1981. "Accumulated Stress of Life Changes and Interpersonal Effectiveness in the Family." *Family Relations* 30:367–371.

Magrabi, F. and W. Marshall. 1965. "Family Developmental Tasks: A Research Model." *Journal of Marriage and the Family* 27:454–461.

McCubbin, H., M. McCubbin, J. Patterson, A. E. Cauble, L. Wilson, and W. Warich. 1983. "CHIP — Coping Health Inventory for Parents: An Assessment of Parental Coping Patterns in the Care of the Chronically Ill Child." *Journal of Marriage and the Family* 45:359–370.

McCubbin, H. and D. Olson. 1984. "Beyond Family Crisis: Family Adaptation." Presented at the Conference on Families in Disaster, Uppsala, Sweden, (June).

Patterson, J. 1985. "Critical Factors Affecting Family Compliance with Home Treatment for Children with Cystic Fibrosis." *Family Relations* 34:79–89.

Patterson, J. and H. McCubbin. 1984. "Gender Roles and Coping." *Journal of Marriage and the Family* 46:95–104.

Pratt, C., V. Schmall, S. Wright, and M. Cleland. 1985. "Burden and Coping Strategies of Caregivers to Alzheimer's Patients." *Family Relations* 34:27–33.

Terkelson, K. 1980. "Toward a Theory of the Family Life Cycle." In E. Carter and M. McGoldrick, eds. *The Family Life Cycle: A Framework for Family Therapy*. New York: Gardner Press, pp. 21–52.

PART 2

---

*Problems of Childhood
and Adolescence*

Facilitation of Mourning During Childhood*

Gilbert Kliman

The Center for Preventive Psychiatry (White Plains, New York), from which this presentation stems, was created to assist adults and children in dealing with situational stresses and strains, so that the maximal degree of health and emotional growth could occur despite severe emotional burdens. Among the over 1000 persons who have come to the Center since it opened 12 years ago, many have been victims of severe, sudden crises not involving object loss. Some have been children who were sexually molested, or who had been badly beaten, or who had witnessed murders in their families. Some have been involved in highly overstimulating experiences, such as romantic involvement with adults of the same sex, or incestuous relations within their own families. Some have been severely ill physically. Some have been in mass disasters such as floods or tornadoes.

No patients have, however, attracted more of our systematic professional interest and consumed more of our professional energies than adults and children who suffer the sudden and then chronic strains of object loss. Never a momentary injury, loss of a loved person, we maintain, is often a long-enduring pathogenic influence. It deserves preventive intervention whenever the loss has occurred early in life, and especially when the early loss is that of the child's parent.

From its beginning, the Center has been interested in helping healthy orphans in order to develop techniques of primary prevention of mental illness. Data concerning a series of 18 untreated orphans show that, as far as neurotic symptomatology goes, not many orphans are free of important symptoms. Nor does the Center for Preventive Psychiatry find that orphans referred even very shortly after bereavement and for purposes said by the family to be preventive are in fact often free of symptoms. Of the children on whom we

*The contributions of Daniel Feinberg, M.D., Betty Buchsbaum, Ph.D., Ann S. Kliman, M.A., Harriet Lubin, M.S.W., Doris Ronald, Florence Herzog, and Myron Stein, M.D., to the preparation of this chapter are gratefully acknowledged.

can report some details today, the Center found the majority were already suffering recognizable symptoms of neurosis, and in some cases, psychosis. We have a growing impression that orphanhood is indeed a categorical damage from which children may successfully recover untreated, but that is also true of fractures of the bone. Apparently a break in a love relationship early in childhood usually needs help in healing. It is our position that means for healing such fractures in a child's love-life are extraordinarily undeveloped, little used and, indeed, shunned.

This chapter is essentially practical in its orientation to technique, describing several forms of treatment of bereaved children, with a minimum of theoretical essay. Probably the best definition of "mourning" for our current purposes is, "the totality of reaction to the loss of a loved object." We omit from this definition any immediate consideration of whether mourning can occur at various stages in childhood, and if so, to what extent one or another investigator judges it has occurred, although such consideration is worthy of volumes. To simplify the task somewhat, because it is actually of extreme complexity, Freud's (1915) definition of the work of mourning will be used, with no detailed reference at this time to the more modern contributions such as those of Bowlby (1960).

Since considerable review of literature on childhood mourning, including the few clinical cases reported in the literature in any detail, has been made elsewhere by this author (Kliman, 1968), a repetition will be avoided here.

It is assumed that the statistical work of Beck (1963), Barry (1960). Kliman (1968), Gregory (1965), and others amply demonstrates the long-standing common-sense impression of many clinicians working with children that death of a parent is a severe insult to psychological health. Especially when bereavement occurs during early childhood, there is an excessive incidence of psychopathology within a few months, and it endures noticeably throughout adult life. These matters have been well established, using exquisitely controlled and anterospective and retrospective series of nonbereaved children and adults from comparable social, ethnic, racial and economic strata. Therefore, we maintain there is much society and the individual have to gain by carefully attending to the problems of each orphan in the adaptation to his loss. Furthermore, the readily detected nature of this pathogenic factor makes it a prime target for the all-too-little developed field of preventive psychiatry.

Deutsch's studies (1937) suggest that the problem, amidst all its kaleidoscopic complexities, includes excessive childhood defensiveness against the emotion of grief. This is especially pernicious when the child's grief is for a dead parent, and his defensiveness against affective charge may become a life-long pathogenic style for a bereaved child. To the extent that Deutsch has correctly discerned a major etiologic component in the emotional disorders following bereavement, one major part of the preventive task is to facilitate mourning by helping release a bereaved child's grief, including sad yearning feelings and associated memories. This must be done in a fashion compatible with the child's defensive repertoire, his developmental state, and his life framework. Then he can experience further development and avoid fixation to the psychosexual stage at which the damaging loss occurred.

The illustrations of mourning facilitation we will now provide are gathered mainly from orphaned children treated with varying degrees of intensity at the Center for Preventive Psychiatry over the past few years. An interesting fact in itself is that our Center now averages at least one such referral every month. There is preventive value in the community's recognition that bereaved children need special help soon and that a place exists where such help can appropriately and congenially be obtained. The children referred have ranged in age from infancy to 18 years and were bereaved for periods of a few hours to as long as five years before coming to the Center. Most of the treated orphans were already symptomatic by the time they reached us. Some of the children were known to the therapist before the parental death occurred, so that some baseline knowledge was obtained. We can also draw upon another source of information about childhood bereavement — our work with dying children and their siblings. Preparing one child's two older sisters for the impending death and then facilitating their adaptation to the actual loss is the subject of one section of this report. Special attention is given in another section to facilitation of feminine identity development in the case of a maternally bereaved girl. Still another section provides data concerning the interrelationships of mourning problems with the multiply determined symptoms of memory impairment in a paternally bereaved boy, thus casting light on the statistically widespread problems of intellectual inhibitions among bereaved children by an in-depth study of an illustrative case.

We will now present a brief survey of the techniques already in use at the Center, moving from customary techniques to those less customary.

PARENT GUIDANCE

Nothing can be more critical to the mourning work of a child than the mourning work of the adults around him and their attitudes toward his work. A major part of the preventive and therapeutic task can often be efficiently focused on parent guidance. Because such guidance techniques are widely practiced and well-known, we will not dwell on them in this survey except for some insufficiently appreciated and essential points.

Parent guidance in cases of childhood bereavement should include at least some check on the possibility that the parent may be out of synchronization with the very difficult mourning rhythms of his or her child. Forceful evidence of such dysrhythmia within a family is often found when a widow is ready to remarry, particularly if her remarriage is planned for a year or less after bereavement. She may need assistance to realize that her children are much slower than she to give up the lost object, because of their greater defensiveness in permitting the work of mourning to proceed. During latency, mourning is apt to be particularly silent and slow. Throughout childhood, the tardy pace with which the old object is decathected is one cause of the poor acceptance of substitute parents. It is one factor which accounts for the otherwise surprisingly higher incidence of certain psychopathology, Gregory's large-scale study reports (1965). Among families where the parent has remarried, there is actually a higher incidence of truancy, school failure and school dropout than among families where the surviving parent remains single. We must take these unpleasant facts very seriously, as they come from indisputable anterospective study over a decade with 10,000 school children. The unmistakable implication is that we must guide parents preventively to help their bereaved children with utmost tact when a remarriage is impending. At this juncture, however, our sketch of technique need not dwell on what is already common practice.

The surviving parent also needs guidance and support to avoid surprisingly regular tendencies to use the child as a partial replacement for the lost spouse. Our series of 18 nonpatient orphans (A. Kliman, 1968) showed that seven out of eight families had one child who was chosen as bed companion for the surviving parent. Nine out of these 18 untreated orphans began a pattern of bed-sharing with the surviving parent. This occurred in families which had no previous pattern of inter-generation bed-sharing. A six-year follow-up showed that the tendency, generally manifest within a few weeks after bereavement, continues to be a major one. It is unquestionably an obstacle to full mourning, in the sense of moving on to healthy substitutes for the lost object. One of the initial study's bed-sharers, then age 11, by age 17 was over six feet tall. He had an active adolescent heterosexual life, but still shared the mother's bed several times a week!

Since a large fraction of bereaved children become parent bed-sharers, we can speculate reasonably that the incestuous impulses of many bereaved children — particularly when the bereavement is of the same sex parent — are a major obstacle to the progress of mourning. To mourn and be thereby freed for the loving of other persons is dangerous when the most available other person is the surviving opposite sex parent who is also a tempting bed partner.

Bed-sharing is, of course, only one form of erotically tinged distortion of parent-child interaction after a death in the family. One sixteen-year-old girl, who began treatment two weeks after the death of her mother from breast carcinoma, found herself in severe strain. She had been rather circumspect about undressing in front of her father, so long as her mother was alive. Now she was inclined to experiment with her father's reactions when walking around in her bra and panties. She wanted to check on whether her new behavior increased the frequency with which he displayed a nervous fly-touching mannerism. In this case, the child's developmental status permitted interpretation of her own erupting yearnings for closeness to the surviving parent via assumption of her mother's sexual role. Simultaneously, guidance of her father in providing the still necessary circumspection and structuring of his interactions with the excited girl permitted her to enter a vigorous and affectively profuse preoccupation with memories of her mother. Mourning was to that extent facilitated, because it was less dangerous to decathect the lost mother when the child's superego could be supported as the mother had once made possible.

A CASE OF LEARNING INHIBITION AND MEMORY DISTURBANCE RELATED TO PATHOGENIC MOURNING

Continuing with work which is often done well in any psychoanalytically-oriented, multidisciplinary setting, we come now to one of the most familiar problems of bereaved children—a combination of intellectual disinterest, learning difficulties, and disturbances in the field of memory. Such bereaved children are to be found in every grade school, out of proportion to their expected frequency of bereavement, among underachievers. Their treatment can be modeled on a standard psychotherapy, but in order to be successful, special factors must be considered, some of which are clearly seen in the following material.

The case of Richard (a patient of Dr. Betty Buchsbaum's) was selected to illustrate, first, that the patient could engage in a process similar to that of mourning in the course of weekly psycho-analytically-oriented psychotherapy sessions over a period of 16 months. It also appeared likely that the therapeutic facilitation of mourning helped neutralize the patient's impaired, conflicted memory sphere, freeing it for further development.

The patient had been referred at the age of 8 for treatment because of failing grades, inattention and restlessness at school. Immaturity and a tendency to forget what he was about to do were noted by his mother to have become exaggerated following the death of his maternal grandfather the summer before. The grandfather's death was the last of a series of separations and losses experienced by Richard. Early in his infancy, his mother had been briefly hospitalized because of phlebitis. When he was 4½ years of age, his father was discovered to have lung cancer and underwent surgery. During the following year, the cancer metastasized to the brain and Richard's father died. During the course of the next two years, the patient's older brother married and moved to another state, while his sister left for an out-of-town college. Richard's mother had returned to college, obtained a Master's degree and worked at a position that required occasional out-of-town travelling.

The patient impressed us as an alert-looking, articulate and socially responsive boy. His initial sessions communicated a sense of restlessness with an apparent nonchalance and bravado that barely concealed his anxiety and tension. He believed treatment had been recommended because he was "mixed up a lot," and did things such as learning a spelling word and then forgetting it. He revealed he even forgot how to spell his name when he was in first grade. Other references to forgetting included not knowing when his mother was due to leave for or return from a trip. A relationship between object loss and the loss of information was suggested by Richard's concern that a classmate, on whom he depended for information, might not be in his class the following years.

Another prominent symptom related to his memory difficulty occurred in the form of "slips of the tongue." Those slips tended to be more closely bound to references to illness and death than was the more general forgetting phenomenon. Thus, Richard referred to an ambulance as an "alabance." Again, when describing a game he used to play with his father, he used the word "internal" instead of air terminal.

There was also evidence that when Richard did recall emotionally significant content, he did so in a rather primitive and immature mode. Remembering was often achieved in a visually-oriented context rather than through verbal expression. The tendency to use relatively primitive mechanisms to deal with memories was considered a function of the strength of the affects still attached to the ideas so expressed. The phenomenon included relatively benign events such as projecting onto a tree branch outside the office window the notion of a man's arm. Once, Richard was momentarily confused when he almost misidentified a man who resembled his father and thought the man to be his father.

Richard also reported that he occasionally saw things as appearing smaller and more distant than they were, as well as larger and closer. He then associated the feeling of distance to the notion of people leaving or dying. In the following session, his comments led the therapist to speculate about his desire for his father to be alive again. Richard revealed that he had actually hallucinated his father, who had appeared as a "very small man in the kitchen cabinet." This hallucination had occurred the previous year, with Richard's awareness of its imaginary nature. It would seem those thoughts and memories which were still too intensely cathected to be considered in a rational, secondary process mode could be allowed expression in the visual sphere, where hopes and wishes might still be concretely experienced.

Let us now examine the proposition that the mourning occurred, that fantasies and memories associated with his father's death were gradually worked over, partially decathected, and usefully reassimilated by Richard. In addition, let us see if this mourning work did facilitate a reorganization and further growth of the memory sphere.

Richard's references to his father's death were initially expressed via personally remote, destructive, and elaborately dramatized fantasies. Man-crushing trucks and explosive fires were among the prominent instruments of death. By the fifth month of treatment, and no doubt significantly following a vacation from treatment, there was a marked reduction in explosive and destructive themes. Richard began to express fears about his mother's welfare and disclosed dreams and thoughts about monsters. Simultaneously, he began to describe detailed memories of the course of his father during the terminal illness and death.

Games such as checkers and block-play elicited a growing number of associations and increasingly distinct reminiscences concerning his father's activities before his illness. Details about his physical deterioration were repeatedly described with increasing clarity, as with a blurred image coming into focus. Finally, in the 37th session, Richard spontaneously listed all the things he could recall about his father. His inventory included the fact that everyone in his family was sad at the funeral. This reference was Richard's first attempt to admit his own unhappiness. The fear of his inability to control his sadness was reflected in the next session when he created a story about a boy who flooded his home with his tears. The boy attempted to cover his eyes but then tears escaped from his ears and mouth. When the boy stopped up these openings, he experienced such pressure that he thought he would crack up. Then Richard went on to tell how the boy left home because of the flooding and cried for 200 years, flooding a complete desert. An Indian shot the boy for ruining the ground with his tears. In view of these associations to sadness, Richard's comment that remembering his father's illness "just causes trouble" is only too understandable.

Six weeks later, Richard was able to explain that he could now remember well enough but did not report his memories because doing so "would get him down." Concomitantly, he demonstrated his excellent skill in playing "Concentration," a memory game. It was considered to be more than a coincidence that on this same day Richard complained that he did not see why he was in treatment since the therapist could not bring back his father. The patient was reluctantly relinquishing hope for his father's return. In doing so, the incipient expression of the mourning process was further advanced. Richard's ego had entered into the task that Freud described as severing its "attachment to the non-existent object" (Freud, 1917). As he did so, he could go on to enjoy exhibiting his memory in the context of the concentration game. Reality gratifications now began to compete more successfully for Richard's attention.

A major part of the treatment work concentrated on transference reactions. When he felt abandoned by the therapist because of a temporary break in treatment, he literally perceived the therapist as very far away, although the seating arrangement was unchanged. The perceptual illusion reversed when the underlying sensitivity to loss was genetically interpreted, ultimately with reference to the father's and grandfather's deaths.

In support of the speculation that Richard could devote his energies more directly to the demands of his environment are the following data. After the first year in treatment, his reading ability rose from a first to third-grade level. His teacher reported improvement in executing his assignments and increased interests in science and social studies projects. Comparison of WISC scores obtained after 16 months of treatment revealed a Full Scale I.Q. gain of 12 points. The three subtests contributing most to the increment were Comprehension, Similarities, and Picture Arrangement. The findings suggested an improved ability to conceptualize verbally and to deal more meaningfully with social interactions. At home, too, Richad became more cooperative and independent. In addition, an element of enthusiasm replaced the avoidance usually evoked by school assignments.

The lifting of constriction and increased independence and sociability were equally evident. Richard's growing capacity to face and undertake the work of mourning is believed to be a significant factor in his increasingly successful engagement in memory-related tasks. Richard seemed no longer required to use his memory as a wish-dominated vehicle which held on to his father's image. Rather, as he began to acknowledge and master his overwhelming experiences of pain, anger and sadness, he was able to register the daily events of his life and participate in them with freedom and even pleasure.

WHEN A SIBLING DIES

Here we move further into uncommonly encountered or sought after technical problems. The Center has worked with a small number of children who experienced recent sibling bereavement or were seen in advance of such an experience. In one family, Charles was dying of leukemia. His treatment in The Cornerstone Project has been described elsewhere (Kliman, 1968). A principal feature of his work was that he emerged from a state of regressed clinging to his mother at age 4½, a state which had been precipitated six months earlier by his initial hospitalization for leukemia. He had begun experiencing feminine impulses and transvestist tendencies, with girlishness of gait, voice and mannerisms. It was impressive that, as he was able to talk very frankly with the analyst about reality matters, these severe psychological symptoms cleared entirely. The Cornerstone personnel were particularly moved by the child's ability to state that he knew he was going to die. We were sustained in our own anticipatory grief by the fact that the child's new-found ability to make such truthful statements was associated with marked clinical improvement and strengthening of his character.

At age 6, Charles died in the hospital. To the end, he maintained a matter-of-fact assertive attitude toward his own medical management, including even the ultimate moment of his death.

He kept realistic watch over his oxygen supply, and on two occasions noticed when it was deficient, calling attention to his own vital needs to make sure they were cared for. As he gasped his last breath he was with his mother, to whom he said: "Mommy, I think I'm dying now. You better call the doctor."

We were all fortified by the astonishing ability of this at first weak little boy to face the reality of his own death. Now we wish to report preventive work which was done simultaneously with his sisters.

Charles had two sisters, Barbara and Carol. At the time his leukemia was first diagnosed, they were 6 and 8. Both sisters were relatively healthy emotionally despite their brother's problems, and despite the fact that their burdens were magnified by marital discord and a divorce. Their parents' divorce occurred just as Charles' leukemia was discovered. At that time, Carol developed a transient symptom, while Charles was still in the hospital for diagnosis. She began to pilfer from family members. Several psychotherapy interviews cleared the problem. But two years later, the mother agreed that preventive intervention was desirable for both girls, despite their continuing good functioning. The mother was in guidance and therapy herself, not for this essay's purposes, little will be described of that important task.

It was decided that during Charles' terminal months, both sisters would be treated by one therapist.* Preventive treatment for both girls, who were interviewed separately, could be categorized from at least five points of view insofar as the initiation of mourning occurred. These were, first, active forthrightness by the therapist; second, a stimulation of "immunizing" discussions when material was ripe; third, direct encouragement of catharsis, fourth, recurring emphasis on reality; fifth, direct encouragement of affective components of mourning.

Both Barbara and Carol were *dealt with forthrightly* from the outset. The relation of their presence at the Center to the seriousness of their brother's illness was elicited from them early. A dialogue then ensued about the physical details of Charles' condition. In Carol's treatment, this forthrightness led to much discussion of the previous deaths of pets, and her own advice that children are less upset about such events if they are told the truth right away.

Immunizing discussions were conducted, in the sense that the imminent loss was affectively experienced in small doses by discussions of the previous deaths of animals and people known, but not emotionally important to the girls. As they brought up such material, the slightest reference to Charles was underlined by the therapist. The girls had experienced the death of several cats, dogs and goldfish. Sadness was evoked, and sometimes there were reproaches for mistreatment of the animals. Barbara, who with her lesser tolerance for sadness, also tended to projections of any guilt, bitterly accused her sister of having played aggressively with the family's dog shortly before it died. There was clear echoing of this guilt and sadness-laden theme in a later session concerning reproaches to the sister for similar aggressive play with Charles. With small doses of guilt and sadness being liberated, the two sisters gradually became freer to complain about their mother's neglect of them in favor of Charles.

Catharsis should ideally be both full and controlled, so that a child need not undergo severe regression under the load of affect. Carol felt a temptation to become like Charles and complain about physical pains, experiencing this temptation strictly at a fantasy and discussion level. She had good insight into her desire for more of her mother's attention. She also became aware, with the therapist's interpretation, of a wish that Charles would die and get the family's suffering over with. This expression of death wish was well balanced by an awareness of her affection for Charles and desire for him to get better. Much work was done to help the girls realize the developmental appropriateness of having opposite feelings about one person. Barbara's catharsis was more of angry feelings, but also of sadness, with many thoughts of vengeful ghosts apparently representing projected *angry* impulses mixed with sad ones. One

---

*Daniel Feinberg, M.D. This work has been reported more extensively in "Preventive Therapy with Siblings of a Dying Child," *Journal of the American Academy of Child Psychiatrists*, Vol. 9, October, 1970.

aspect of the work was to encourage the girls to stay with and not run away from their feelings during treatment. It was hoped that this would help strengthen the ego's power to bind painful affects. This is a maneuver independent of the interpretation of the affect, and may be regarded as an exercise in defense-strengthening or tolerance-building somewhat like immunization. When the maneuver was performed, some higher level defensive manifestations were noted in Carol particularly. By the end of one session, she showed signs of strong sublimative interests involving rescue fantasies and becoming a scientist who could cure diseases.

Reality orientation, the fourth of the five categories to be touched on in this summary of the girls' treatment, was oriented especially to the details of Charles' condition. The therapist attempted not only to help the girls report their own perceptions of changes in Charles, but also to understand the emotional reactions of others in the family to these changes. The emotional climate in the family was a matter to which the girls needed to adapt, and the therapist used every clue.

Barbara was less able than Carol to report her perceptions. Carol observed subtle changes in Charles, whom she described as "skinnier . . . his eyes looked like they were out . . . they weren't really out, but they looked bigger." With Barbara, who used avoidance of reality detail quite strongly in her session, the therapist was gently persistent. He was especially careful and especially persistent when Charles actually died. At that time, the concern was that Barbara might make the event unreal or dream-like, and an effort was therefore made to have Barbaa exert mastery by actively recounting all she could of what she knew and had experienced, an effort to which she was able to respond collaboratively.

With Carol, much work was done on a more abstract kind of reality orientation, concerned with the finiteness of life. In the final three months of Charles' life, Carol gradually softened her wishes for her own infinite survival, and began describing finite lives. At the same time, she began speaking of the uselessness of Charles' medication, and how they were being discontinued, as well as how Charles was growing sicker.

The fifth category, *direct encouragement of the work of mourning*, had many aspects. Partly, it consisted of establishing an atmosphere in which memories were an encouraged subject of discussion. Partly, it had occurred in a displaced way through affective discharges over other losses. A therapeutic alliance was easier for the older sister in this regard. Barbara's lesser maturity led to more avoidance and conscious suppression of remembering and feeling sad. Some of the appropriate affects were expressed by displacement into the transference. She was very somber in the session just before Charles' funeral was held. She lingered in the office and would not budge when it came time to leave. The lingering was interpeted as related to how hard it would be to say "gooddbye" to Charles the next day, to someone whom she loved very much, and that all kinds of saying goodbye were hard. Barbara then remained still more sadly and quietly in her chair, and said that she had cried after hearing of Charles' death, and had been thinking of Charles as he died. When the therapist interpreted that some goodbyes and some remembering can take a long time, and crying can happen from time to time afterwards, or sadness without crying, the child was finally able to move, although with hesitation. She was apparently in the throes of depression, with vegetative signs in the sense of locomotor retardation.

Carol was more open, frequently crying tears with her family, frequently bringing up specific memories of Charles' life. She brought the therapist pictures of her brother. A month after the funeral, she reported that she still got sad, but did not cry any more, in fact did not think she could cry even if she wanted to.

Barbara's defensiveness was more rigid, and she would often spend part of her sessions looking out the office window at events on the streets. Her last session, as reported by Dr. Feinberg, is noteworthy in respect to ability to suspend the defensiveness:

> She became quite depressed when I pointed out how hard it was for children to look at what was happening inside them because it might hurt a lot. At this point she began to give forth one memory after another about Charles, finally describing how neighborhood kids had trampled down some of Charles' flowers recently and how they all had died. Saddening a little as she recollected, she added that the flowers would probably grow out again because the seeds were still in the ground. She would plant an onion and watch it grow. I reflected to her about how nice a wish it was that Charles' flowers grow back again and that people also have wishes that brothers who die could also grow back again or be alive again just the way flowers might. She immediately corrected me and said, "No, not like a flower, like a tree." I said that one of the reasons she might want to grow that onion was to express her wish that Charles could have kept on growing. . . and didn't have to stop. She replied, "I never thought of it like that before."

MOURNING AND FACILITATION OF FEMININE IDENTIFICATION IN A MATERNALLY BEREAVED GIRL

Here we find a problem not uncommonly encountered in child treatment centers, but seldom sufficiently thought through. Marie Bonaparte, who grew up motherless, has described the multiform consequences extensively (Bonaparte, 1950). We have had the opportunity to treat several maternal orphans who were girls and therefore severly burdened in the development of their own sexuality.

We first saw Norma, (treated by Harriet Lubin, M.S.W.) then 10½, over five years after her mother had died. It proved feasible, nevertheless, to induce some long overdue mourning. Norma then came to grips with developmental tasks which had been retarded in apparent consequence of the earlier strains. The precipitating problems leading Norma to treatment were episodes of physical complaints appropriately recognized by her father and stepmother as hysterical manifestations. These included generalized warm body feelings, trembling, tingling sensations in all extremities, and inordinate clinging to her stepmother whom she repeatedly asked, "Do you love me?" Norma was under-achieving in school, hesitant and slow in speech, sparse in vocabulary, and desirous of being a nun so that she would not marry. Her peer social life was constricted. History revealed there had been many predisposing or copathogenic experiences prior to the mother's death due to carcinoma of the pancreas. The death occurred rapidly over a one-month period following diagnosis. At that time, the mother was in the first trimester of her fifth pregnancy. There were already three other children living besides Norma. The embryo did not survive. Not only was Norma's father shocked and grief-stricken and withdrawn from Norma, but the child was also burdened by place-ment in the care of an aunt and uncle who were harsh and inconsistent. Four-teen months later, the father married a widow who herself had a large family so that there were ten children in the amalgamated household. Furthermore, a year later, when Norma was almost 8, a cherished maternal uncle died in an automobile crash. He plunged off an eroded embankment in his automobile and his body was never recovered from the river below. When Norma was 9, her father was threatened with the possible loss of business opportunity, and it was in this setting of his continued preoccupation with business difficulties that her presenting complaints arose.

From the beginning, the parents were told that the focus of the treatment was to enable Norma to have more confidence in her thoughts and feelings so that she would not lead such a socially isolated life, nor approach adulthood so frightened of being a woman.

Following an introductory, supportive phase of approximately three months, in which she was seen weekly, the therapeutic alliance and focus with the child and her family moved to the bereavement. From the third month on, Norma's treatment involved her questioning about, remembering, and missing people she had loved and lost, especially her first mother and her uncle. She expressed happy and sad affects appropriately, focusing on the past, the present, and their connections. External events were usefully dwelled upon. They included separations from the therapist for the patient's and for the therapist's vacations, many cancelled or missed appointments, two anniversaries of the first mother's death, and the first anniversary of the hysterical episode. Other interpreted loss reactions were at the anniversary of beginning treatment. Termination was planned seven months ahead. During that period, the child brought the therapist fantasies and misperceptions, using her as a nidus for her crystallizing attempts to identify with an adult woman's life. Transference envy, curiosities and jealous reactions were identified and interpreted as pertaining to the unresolved guilty oedipal relationship to the mysterious, increasingly remembered first mother and to the present mother. Connections were made through the transference reactions to experiences and misunderstandings of the past. Present intellectual misunderstandings were connected to their fore-runners in confusing periods of early childhood. Feminine identification grew, and from wishing to be childless, Norma began a mild, then vivid, interest in heterosexual escapades acceptable to her family. Her gait, dress, voice and interests became those of a fully girlish early adolescent.

Phenomena of the last session are of special interest. The patient developed and recovered from an interpreted amnesia concerning the date of termination. She mastered a dread of saying goodbye, which was interpreted genetically in terms of her mother's death as a goodbye. She became aware of a curious uneasiness about looking up at the building in which the therapist's office was located — a phenomenon related to her waving goodbye to her dying mother in the upper floors of a hospital. At last, in the very last session, there emerged a major connection between being feminine and dying. It emerged as a last-minute, never before expressed question, just in time to be clarified: "Did my mother die because she was having a baby?"

THE SPECIAL PROBLEMS OF DOUBLE ORPHANS

Proceeding further into seldom explored areas of bereavement research, our experience with double orphans is illuminating. Their immediate grief tends to be open, in the literal sense of prolonged anguished crying. Conscious feelings of grief also attend later remembering of the dead parents, more openly and more frequently than with orphans bereaved of one parent. Although causally different, the phenomonologic situation of double orphans is like that of Bender's (1954) psychotic orphans, who grieved profusely and even wildly. The double orphans, like psychotic children, lack adequate defenses. But the lack is in proportion to the great quantity of affect being stimulated by the double loss rather than because of the intrinsic deficiency of defense. Or, we could say the proportional relationship of affect to defense is disturbed by excess over the "average expectable" life strain rather than by the inadequacy of their defenses due to any disease. But the double orphans may also have suffered some actual weakening or exhaustion of defense due to the first loss, on which the second loss is now heaped. The task with double orphans is, therefore, how to facilitate the management of extraordinary quantities of affect becoming detached from two major objects, and specifically how to manage this task without the development of gross deformities and breaches in the testing of perception and in the adaptation to new objects.

One of the double orphans whom we treated would frequently hallucinate. This was a major presenting problem, although in follow-ups he was not apparently psychotic. One task with this four-year-old boy was to provide interpretations to produce a framework of insight, so that he could understand the nature of his hallucinations, especially their wishful, loneliness-induced origin. In a twelve-year-old double orphan, a main accomplishment was to allow more boldness in his adaptation to peer social objects. His high dose of affectively charged conscious memories of both parents became more manageable when catharsis occurred repeatedly in twice-a-week sessions over a ten-week period. For one post-bereavement year, his love-life had been confirmed to going over the parental memories, morbidly pouring over photo albums, prolongedly weeping silent tears of regret for the now idealized life he and his parents had had together. After catharsis in treatment, the mournful ruminations diminished and social life increased, apparently using the now more available libido.

THE CORNERSTONE PROJECT

Before discussing this most unusual of our techniques with bereaved children, a fascinating technique for mourning facilitation developed and used with adults in Mexico is helpful to mention as an introduction. Remus-Araico (1965) has reported excellent results with a series of 12 adult analysands orphaned during childhood. They generally suffered from repressed sad affect and fixation to developmental stages at which the childhood bereavement had occurred, with evidence of a "traumatic neurotic" process. Not only do Remus-Araico's data confirm and enrich the finding of Fleming and her coworkers (1963) in Chicago, they also provide an interesting innovative contribution to the facilitation technique. That contribution is in the form of what Remus-Araico calls "timeless interviews." He found it very useful to arrange that several times during the course of analysis he would meet with the patient for an interview of a duration limited only by the interest and willingness of the patient and analyst. These interviews, which frequently endured several hours, induced a state of remembering with extremely intense detail and high charge of emotion. Remus-Araico frequently felt that the analyst and patient "were standing at the side of the grave together." We believe that such cathartic remembering is indeed difficult to facilitate in adults as well as in children. Yet, to some extent, it appears feasible even in children of preschool age, as well as those who are older. A necessary condition is a positive transference and ample time in which to set the mental stage.

One of the techniques used at the Center involves working 15 hours a week with orphans (and other young patients) in a preventively-oriented nursery school, where the analyst is present in the classroom for six of those hours. This technique appears powerful and has been used for neurotic and psychotic children, as well as to give psychological aid to orphans of preschool age. While the teachers conduct educational activities, the analyst works right in the congenial and communication-evocative classroom setting. He transacts with one child and then moves on to work with another, and then another. In this setting, he is able to interpret material the children express to teachers or to each other, as well as the play and verbal communications made directly to him. When the analyst leaves the classroom after an hour and a half of work each morning, the six or eight child patients who constitute the class remain at work with their teachers.

The teachers are well-trained specialists in early childhood education, working under the analyst's supervision, as well as the supervision of an educational director (Mrs. Doris Ronald). They observe and cultivate, but do not interpret the communications of the children made after the analyst leaves. Thus, while the classroom work continues for the remaining hours of the morning, many fantasies and playful expressions set in motion by the interpretive work of the first 90 minutes continue to emerge and are later reported to the children's analyst. At the same time, these expressions are channeled into ego-building social and educational activities.

We have now worked with about 110 children by this method and are preparing a documentation of the procedure demonstrating that many essential features of a regular child analysis tend to occur despite the unorthodox setting. With the orphans among our Cornerstone patients, a considerable amount of vivid, affectively expressive and ideationally rich energetic mourning work takes place. We mean to include in this emphatic statement all elements of Freud's *Mourning and Melancholia* (1917) definition, the working over of ideas and affects associated with the lost object, the cathecting and decathecting of the mental representative of that object, testing fo the reality of the object's permanent absence, increased identification with the lost object, and use of liberated cathexis for investment in new objects (Freud, 1917).

Time and time again, in the Cornerstone Project's daily sessions with orphans, we find that the child's feelings and thoughts about the analyst are clearly and continuously linked to thoughts, memories and feelings about the dead parent. Even thoughts about extremely frightening and shocking experiences in the past can emerge in the classroom setting, as part of the transference-linked working over. An example is provided by Quentin, a five-year-old who was alone with his father in a car when the father had a heart attack and died in the boy's solitary presence. Quentin entered the Cornerstone Project about six months later, and the following excerpt from his work shows some of the interplay between the pathogenic past and the transference present:

> Quentin went to a great deal of trouble to pull the analyst's beard, and made a drawing of the analyst with a very long beard. The analyst was required to help, and to depict Quentin going for a ride on the analyst's beard, straddling the beard. Quentin then began playing automobile riding games and speaking of his father. He placed some paint in a bowl of water and said it reminded him of blood, saying, "This is very dangerous. It's my daddy's blood." Continuing to develop the blood theme, Quentin thought about how the blood in a person's heart could stop moving and then a scientist could stick the person in the heart to make it work again. He spoke of good and bad scientists and whether other things besdies caterpillars could go into a cocoon and come out butterflies.

Up to this point, we can see that the analyst's person, particularly his beard, was transitional in the series that led to his father and thoughts of his father's death and fantasies of metamorphosis or reincarnation. Quentin proceeded to thoughts about cars crashing, wondering if his now late school bus had been in a crash, and what that would sound like. He grew tired, wanted to nap, and draped some play jewels over his head.

They were "the flowers you put on a dead person." Lying very quietly he then said, "Would you be sad if a friend died?", hastening to explain, "I thought my daddy was fooling. I asked the man who came if Daddy was alive or dead, but I thought he was just fooling, but he wasn't."

The next day, Quentin demonstrated a marked continuity of theme in his Cornerstone work, and approached the teacher with the same colored beads, this time announcing, "I'm an angel."

Briefly recapitulating the work of the previous day for Quentin, to let him know of the relevance of this remark, the analyst was then met with further details of the fatal episode: "A man came and pulled me by the shoulders and I cried."

The analyst interpreted that Quentin must have wanted to stay with his daddy, and was still hoping that his daddy was just fooling. The child responded with some further ideas about needles that could start a heart working again, which the analyst interpreted as thoughts which come because it would have been wonderful if Quentin could still have his father living, and Quentin would like to be a person who could have saved his father. In response, Quentin had two sets of thoughts:

> First, Quentin asked if the school could get him an oxygen gauge, which he wanted to keep in the doll house he was now furnishing. Then he spoke of houses which are nice and houses which are not nice; scientists who are good and scientists who are bad. Scientists who are good save people and scientists who are bad keep people tied up.

In later work, this theme of goodness and badness was interpretable in terms of his anger at the father for having left him by dying, and his dread that if the father knew how angry Quentin was, the father would be angry at Quentin. The Cornerstone work proceeded, with increasing clarity of linkage and equation between the father and the male analyst, who was openly loved and died many times in the child's fantasies.

EVOCATION OF YEARINGS FOR AN UNKNOWN FATHER

The opportunity to work with a posthumous child is rare. At the Center, it was approximated by the presence in the school of a child who had suffered the death of his father at several weeks of age. He had never actually known his father and it is of some interest to note the vicissitudes of his work, by means of which he arrived at a useful awareness of what was missing in his life. The presence of a man therapist (Myron Stein, M.D.) within a heterosexual team of constructively collaborating adults, was probably a facilitator of his yearnings. In that emotionally nourishing setting, where his need for a father was to some extent really met by the frequent presence of the analyst, he could dare to let the yearnings emerge. The procedure is, of course, not strictly the same as the work of helping a child mourn for a loved person he has actually known, but is reported because of its relevance to the general problem of childhood bereavement.

David entered the Cornerstone Nursery at the age of three years, five months. Not only had he been paternally bereaved several weeks after birth, but his mother also had a chronic, presumably fatal illness. His two brothers were two and five years older than he.

This was a family in which a great deal of high drama went on, but always in terms of actions, veiled hints, without direct acceptance, recognition of or communication of these matters between the various people. Issues regarding death, separation, being left behind, came up rapidly and in many ways during the first year of David's treatment.

Initially, the matter of separation from the mother arose. This was a mother who wanted to leave immediately, who found it an intolerable burden to have to put in time staying with David in school. She was constantly referring to the issues of being there or not being there, and separation, but always in a displaced fashion, not directly relating it to the bereavement or to her own illness. She would do this with jokes. When David was shy one day, hiding behind his mother's skirts rather than relating directly to the teachers, she made the joke, "I think I left David at home today." This reference to his being elsewhere, not being there or being lost, was repeated in many ways.

We did insist that the mother stay on with David a bit for several weeks rather than abruptly leaving him. During that time, he focused repeatedly on his fear of her leaving. It was possible to point out to him his sadness, his fearfulness, his sudden noninvolvement when she would be away. This was sufficiently helpful so that when his mother did separate he was able to stand it. David's concern about people being sick or away came up with a shocked reaction whenever anyone was ill. If a teacher, a therapist or other children were away, David was very upset, and this upset was also pointed out to him in terms of his being worried about something happening to people. When his mother went for a periodic examination at the hospital, he was also upset and focused on the fear that something would happen to the mother. The therapist discussed the child's awareness of the mother's being followed in the hospital because of an illness, which, however, was being treated and attended to as much as possible. His concern about his own body integrity came up in terms of his worries about his own physical examination, linked to thoughts of his mother.

The actual fact of David's father's being absent and of his missing his father came up for the first time some months after he had been in the nursery. This was a completely avoided subject before then, and when the patient finally brought it up at home, his older brother's reaction was to turn to the mother and say, "Mom, this kid's nuts." In school, David made a magic potion of mud, dirt, water and paint. He was able to express exactly what the magic potion was in terms of, "Magic to bring a father back." He was able to express his loneliness for his father at this point, and his wish for a father as expressed in this magic potion. He built a snowman outside and when a few of the children broke it down, he showed real despondency. He said that this was a real man. The analyst pointed out to him that he wished so much that he could have a real man, like a father, that when his substitute for the real man, namely the snowman, was destroyed, he missed it badly. He was able to agree with and seemed relieved by the interpretation.

There followed a change from his typical way of functioning. Initially, he would behave like a puffed up big little man, talking in a loud voice, denying an anxiety and depression, instigating fights, being like a little sheriff in the classroom. Thereafter, he was able, after admitting his sadness and his missing having a father, to be more of a little boy with a little boy's needing of his father, missing of his father, and sadness about not having his father. There ensued a playing of games with the therapist in which they would eat together, prepare meals together, and trade gold with one another. Much of the work seemed related to his very much longed for process of identification with a father or a male.

Vacations were hard for all the children, as were holidays, and he found them difficult, too, in line with material discussed above. Transference interpretations were made in terms of David having to be tougher, more abusive, and less communicative following and just before vacations and holidays. In response, he showed minimal changes initially, but then more directly demanded the therapist's attention and less directly avoided it.

For a long time, this rough, tough little man had needed to deny positive feelings towards the analyst. He referred to the analyst as stupid or "dootie." After the interpretation of missing the father, wanting to make a father through the magic potion or the snowman, when he was able to become more of a little boy, he was also able to directly express his positive feelings towards the analyst.

TECHNICAL SEPARATION REACTIONS AS FACILITATORS OF MOURNING

In one case treated in the Cornerstone Project, there was an unexpected necessity to suddenly help a child deal with the death of his father. The death occurred as a result of an airplane crash when the child had already been acquainted with the analyst (Gilbert Kliman, M.D.) and the teachers for six weeks prior. He had been attending the Cornerstone school because of problems of transvestism and aggressive behavior. A feature of his immediate reactions to the death of his father was a combination of heightened positive transference with considerable expression of sad affect and yearning for the return of his father. The child made steady clincial progress, overcoming the transvestism and aggressive behavior and experiencing a rather vigorous mourning process, including conscious and unconscious identifications with his father, much remembering associated with sad affect, and a gradual giving up of hopes for the father's return. Throughout the treatment process, a major feature was close attachment to the male analyst, as well as female teachers. In retrospect, it seems that the prolonged presence of a heterosexual team, and especially the many-hours presence of a real male substitute for the lost male parent, permitted the expression of what might otherwise have been an unbearable yearning and sense of emptiness in his life. This child expressed his sadness upon the death of his father both overtly at a conscious level and in multiform unconscious expressions at a level of symbolic, verbal, playful, creative and dream activities. The father's death appeared to increase the intensity of transference to both teachers and the analyst. Simultaneous with passionate attachments to the therapeutic team members, Jay dwelled on thoughts of his lost father, experiencing powerful sadness and increasing identification with the father's traits. His clinical progress was excellent after two years in the school, and he continued working with the analyst twice a week on a regular individual basis thereafter.

His experience when the treatment was to be reduced still further is dramatic evidence of how a bereaved child experiences resonance of treatment separations and loss.

At the end of three years treatment, Jay and the analyst discussed his progress and made plans for a vacation and then reduction of treatment from twice to once a week. At that point, Jay, who had been speaking of how well he felt he was doing in school and socially, experienced a momentary loss of balance, as he was perched on a worktable, reaching up to a high shelf. He became frightened that he was to fall, and the analyst moved over toward him, saying that this was a way of letting us know that he still needed help with his accident trouble, which he had been talking about quite a bit lately. Jay said that it sure was a trouble that he needed help with. In a few moments, Jay said he was frightened because he was seeing "a dark shadow man" in the doorway, adding, "I think I'm having hallucinations. I get this feeling when I look into a dark room or a closet, or I walk by a doorway, the feeling that I'm seeing a dark shadow man in there — a scary man." Jay and the analyst then discussed the way this "hallucination" had come up when talking about something that would make Jay lonely for the analyst — not seeing him in his office. At first, Jay denied there was any connection, but then further elaborated his fearfulness, saying that he also sometimes was afraid that he was having hallucinations because on a couple of occasions he thought he was seeing flying saucers — once at night and once in the middle of a foggy day. Again the analyst reminded Jay of the connection previously established to lonely feelings and outer space monsters, a connection which at first Jay denied by saying that the fears had started before his father died, and they also came on when he did not feel lonely. Later he said it was funny though, that it had come on when talking about not seeing the analyst as often. He would not like that. He wanted to come more often, three times a week, at least twice a week, and not just once a week.

The session ended with Jay's feeling much more relaxed and clearly aware that he feared and resented the reduction in treatment but could tolerate it.

This appears to be an example of transference neurotic process. The hallucinatory experience was precipitated by a separation pending in the form of a vacation to be followed by a reduction in frequency of sessions. There was technical utility in the separation, which could be analyzed in the light of the transference from father to analyst. The symptom of flying saucer and outer space men fears was transferred into the analytic session and appeared specifically in relation to the separation experience, which could thus be better understood by the child because of its narrow framework.

CORNERSTONE WORK WITH A DOUBLE ORPHAN

Marvin, age four years and six months at onset of treatment, was from an impoverished black family where both parents were physically ill for several years. His mother died of chronic hypertension and a cardiac failure when Marvin was three years and eleven months. His father, who had been a kidney disease invalid and homebound most of Marvin's life, died only one month after the mother.

Compounding the tragic fracturing of Marvin's life had been severe prior stress. Especially pathogenic had been his mother's insidious dementia as she succumbed to hypertension. Becoming a recluse, suspicious of visitors to her sad and increasingly unkempt home, she failed to toilet train her children, who often ran naked and excreted on the floor.

When able to shop, she would leave the children in the care of their weakening, bed-bound, and finally blind father. On one such dreary occasion, Marvin and his one year older sister played with matches under the stove and set a blaze which brought the fire department before any serious damage occurred. Neighbors and firemen who rescued the helpless father and children called the SPCC on finding the floors stewn with old feces.

The deaths occurred a few months later. Marvin's maternal grandmother, freed then from the prohibiting suspicions of her now deceased daughter, came to assume the care of the two children. They were nearly feral wolf-children. Marvin was almost without useful language as well as untrained. Soon enrolled in a day-care center, Marvin was disruptive, restless, and unmanageably aggressive. Referred to Cornerstone, initial examination revealed him to be agitated, incoherent, and anxiously responding to hallucinations seen on the classroom ceiling.

In the first five months at Cornerstone, Marvin continued to hallucinate, and spoke of fire in the ceiling. He gradually became very attached to the analyst, the teachers, and the black handyman. The hallucinations cleared concurrently with completion of the first major interpretative work. This work was that when Marvin began to misidentify the black handyman as his father, the therapist was able gradually to interpret the lonely, wishful quality of the delusion. Marvin was then able to cling physically to the teachers, whom he called "Mother," in contrast to his formerly hostile and disruptive relations to teachers. The availability of new objects to whom Marvin could transfer some of his old investments of love appeared highly useful.

After five months with his first therapist (Myron Stein, M.D.), the project's financial necessities required that two groups be reduced to one. The remaining group had a different analyst (Gilert Kliman, M.D.).

The transition was used with surprising advantage. Marvin insisted that the new analyst was really the first one. It was feasible to point out the similarity of this delusion to the handyman-father delusion. Thereupon Marvin began to speak to his grandmother and sister about how the first doctor "wasn't coming back anymore," and for the first time spoke of his mother and father in this same realistic way. It thus appeared to have been an assimilable experience to lose the first doctor. With the moderate dose of loss, and with a replacement immediately available, improved reality testing was feasible, and further growth occurred.

With the second analyst, obvious questing for the analyst as father occurred, with open anger, sadness and weeping on many days when the analyst would end his 90-minute participation in the classroom procedures. The small daily dose of loss was digestible with the sweetening vehicle of two maternal teachers who remained during and after the analyst left each day. Genetic interpretation of the transference expressions of protests and sadness led to many relevant memories being evoked of Marvin's life with his parents, charged with protest and anguished grief over their absence. The process of identification with some of their now remembered activities and traits was clear. For a while, a feminine identity trend began to hold sway, with powerful yearning to learn to cook in school, dressing in ladies' clothes, speaking of the wonderful pies, cakes and pancakes his mother used to make for him.

At this point a synergism of educational and analytic techniques occurred, as often happens in the Cornerstone situation. The teachers helped Marvin to learn to cook, while the analyst helped him understand his wish to have his mother inside him and to become like her so that he would not be lonely for her. This work led to his falling in love with the teachers, his sister and grandmother, all of whom he wished to marry. He then became very focused on one teacher and one girl in the Cornerstone group, making many gentlemanly and some not so refined romantic overtures and voyeuristic approaches.

Marvin's intellectual development then proceeded vigorously, as he reached the oedipal phase. He now appears nonpsychotic and of good intelligence. After 14 months, he went into a public school. No aspects of his treatment were so important as the dynamic and genetic interpretations of transference separation reactions. Therapeutic induction of mourning occurred through analysis of transference.

DISCUSSION AND CONCLUSION

There is general agreement that the process of mourning, as Freud defined it in *Mourning and Melancholia* (1917), is much more difficult and often much less complete for young children than it is for adolescents and adults. Some believe that successful or complete mourning is not possible until adolescence. We hope we have documented reasons for an optimistic view when intervention occurs to facilitate the process.

We also view optimistically the immediate treatability and analyzability of bereaved children.

In his *Analysis Terminable and Interminable* (1937), Freud emphatically stated that psychoanalysis proceeds most effectively "if the patient's pathogenic experiences belong to the past, so that his ego can stand at a distance from them. In states of acute crisis analysis is to all intents and purposes unusable. The ego's whole interests are taken up by the painful reality and it withholds itself from analysis, which is attempting to go below the surface and uncover the influences of the past" (Freud, 19674).

Many analysts today still believe that adults should not be taken into analysis in the midst of an ongoing love affair, or after the death of a loved person, especially during the period of acute mourning. Anna Freud goes further and suggests that child analysis will be less effective than ordinarily to the degree that "the threat, the attacker or the seducer is a real person, in contrast to situations where the child's fears, fights, crises and conflicts are the product of his inner world" (Freud, 1968).

We would like to present a somewhat different conclusion from the Freuds, although based upon reasoning which is similar up to a point. It is our experience, especially with childen of a very young age, but also with adults and adolescents who have been in acute bereavement situations, that this crisis itself often forces or facilitates the tendency of a person to go below the surface of his daily conscious life and deal inexorably and regressively with influences of the past. The particular crisis of bereavement seems an exceptionally powerful potentiator of the emergence of the past, and therefore, we submit, makes the patient — adult and child alike — unusually available if the therapist is willing to accept the full range of communications brought to him and deal with them unflinchingly as material for scrutiny rather than as reasons to reject the task. Indeed, we would draw the attention of analysis to the exceptionally strong disposition of crisis patients to form strong transferences which develop rapidly and are not only best handled with analytic technique but also can facilitate such an approach.

The flow of love and hate in transference provides an exceptional opportunity for a patient to experience manageable doses of the same emtoions he experienced with love and hate objects in real life outside of treatment. The therapeutic situation, whether by design or not, usually imposes new demands for reaction to loss. When the loss reactions occurring in treatment are deliberately scrutinized and focused upon, a bereaved child has a new chance to work through the reaction to the death of a parent, because the close of transferred reaction is more easily bearable than the original. Because the transferred reaction is subjected to interpretation, the child has an increased repertoire of means at his disposal for mastery, including mourning and going forward with life's new loves and tasks.

In other respects, we are fully in agreement with Anna Freud, who stated (1968) that we still cannot know how far the neglect of developmental needs can be undone by treatment. She apparently includes in this suspension of judgment how far the absence of a parent and its myrid consequences may be undone by treatment. In a situation such as parent loss, she points out, therapists may be unwilling to restrict themselves to analysis and may find other avenues of approach. One such approach is turning the treatment situation itself into an "improved version of the child's initial environment, and within this framework aim at the belated fulfillment of the neglected developmental needs." Another approach is an endeavor to share the work with parents, who may be able to undo some of the harm they have caused. In the Cornerstone Method and in some of our other methods, we have certainly used the first modification to an extent. With some cases, we have added considerable effort to induce a change in the surviving parent's behavior, particularly where fresh pathogenic insult was added to the previous loss. This is true, for example, when a parent begins a dangerously seductive custom.

After so much technical detail, we would like to close on a missionary note. It is our expectation that a great deal more can be done in the prevention of mental illness than has been attempted up to this point. As a profession of healers, we have shown an extraordinary prejudice for the treatment of those who are far advanced in their need for healing. We have used little energy with those who are still under the formative influence of the original damaging forces. The younger a patient is, indeed, the less likely he is to receive our profession's attention.

A prime target for the development of assessable services in the prevention of mental illnesses is any homogeneous early-age group which suffers from a common variable likely to increase the incidence of psychopathology. Such a group can readily be found among bereaved or one-parent children entering nursery, headstart or daycare systems. For this, among other reasons, we emphasize the Cornerstone services as a means to multiply efficiency in use of psychiatric hours, making preventive efforts practical.

We are prepared to go further in missionary zeal and express the opinion that parent guidance has not received adequate scientific opportunity for assessment of effectiveness. It should be assessed in situations likely to yield a very high incidence of pathology in untreated states. We further admit that programs of even more superficial approach, such as parent education without guidance, also have been prematurely written off as hopelessly weak and ineffective.

Unless we systematically explore, control and assess the effectiveness of applied psychoanalytically oriented means for large-scale prevention, we shall have defaulted in using the most obvious measures while immersing ourselves mainly in matters of great professional fascination without great hope of social yield.

So far as our Center's projects for the immediate future are concerned, we are beginning to expand the applications of the Cornerstone Method and its educational and therapeutic derivatives. We also persist in evolving still more widely utilizable procedures, based on psychoanalytic knowledge, but relying less on interpretive techniques. Also, we hope to have control groups answering questions concerning feasibility of prevention. We are now developing a program which will give preventive services to 100 preschool children in situational crises each year. The focus will be on a narrow range of age population, suffering from a few pathogenic factors in common. The assessment problems will be greatly reduced because of the homogeneous age combined with the uniformity of pathogenic variables. Our most likely target group at present seems to be preschool children temporarily placed in foster care, which involves them in a bereavement reaction. It is our belief that some of the best hopes for the future of psychiatry and psychoanalysis lie in such scientific and social opportunities, making efforts to phrase some of our questions in answerable form.

REFERENCES

Barry, H. and E. Lindemann. 1960. "Critical Ages for Maternal Bereavement in Psychoneuroses," *Psychosomatic Medicine*, 22:166.

Beck, A.T., et al. 1963. "Childhood Bereavement and Adult Depression," *Archives of General Psychiatry*, 9:295.

Bender, L. 1954. "Children's Reactions to Death of a Parent," in *A Dynamic Psychopathology of Childhood*. Springfield, Illinois: Charles C. Thomas.

Bonaparte, M. 1950. *Five Copy Books* (1939). London: Imago.

Bowlby, J. 1960. "Grief and Mourning in Infancy." *The Psychoanalytic Study of the Child*, 15:9, New York: International Universities Press.

Deutsch, H. 1937. "Absence of Grief," *Psychoanalytic Quarterly*, 6:12

Fleming, J. 1963. "Activation of Mourning and Growth by Psychoanalysis," *International Journal of Psychoanalysis*, 44:419.

Freud, A. 1968. "Indications and Contraindications for Child Analysis," *The Psychoanalytic Study of the Child*, 22. New York: International Universities Press.

Freud, S. (1917). "Mourning and Melancholia," in J. Strachey (ed.) *The Standad Edition of the Complete Psychological Works of Sigmund Freud*, Vol. 14. London: Hogarth Press, 1957.

Freud, S. (1937). "Analysis Terminable and Interminable," in J. Strachey (ed.). *The Standard Edition of the Complete Psychological Works of Sigmund Freud*, Vol. 23. London: Hogarth Press, 1964.

Furman, R. 1964. "Death of a Six-Year-Old's Mother During His Analysis." *The Psychoanalytic Study of the Child*, 19:377. New York: International Universities Press.

Gregory, I. 1965. "Anterospective Data Following Childhood Loss of a Parent," *Archives of General Psychiatry*, 13:99.

Kliman, G. 1968. *Psychological Emergencies of Childhood*. New York: Grune and Stratton.

Remus-Araico, J. 1965. "Some Aspects of Early-Orphaned Adults' Analyses," *Psychoanalytic Quarterly*, 34:316.

Solnit, A.J. and S. Provence. 1963. *Modern Perspectives in Child Development*. New York: International Universities Press.

Vernick, J. and M. Karon. 1965. "Who's Afraid of Death on a Leukemia Ward?", *American Journal of Diseases of Children*, 109:393.

8

Good Grief: Preventive Interventions for Children and Adolescents

Sandra Sutherland Fox

In the Boston area in one recent year:

- A seventeen-year-old boy begged his teacher and classmates to leave the classroom and then, in the presence of those who remained, shot himself in the head.
- An elementary-school principal committed suicide.
- Three kindergarten youngsters in separate communities were run over and killed by their school buses as they leaned under the wheel to pick up something they had dropped. Two of their mothers witnessed the accidents; in all three accidents, other students were on the bus.
- A seventh-grader went home from school with a headache and died that night of a cerebral hemorrhage.
- A seven-year-old in a residential school for cognitively handicapped children was diagnosed as having cancer of the liver and died two weeks later.
- Three siblings, all of whom attended the same elementary school, were burned to death in a house fire witnessed by many of their classmates who lived in the neighborhood.
- A crossing guard for a parochial elementary school was killed in front of two hundred youngsters when a car driven by a grandfather who was picking up two children from the school ran over her. Two of the crossing guard's grandchildren were in the group of youngsters who witnessed the death.
- An elementary-school psychologist, beloved by the children, died of cancer.

These and many other deaths generated grief and mourning for the families of the victims, but each death also affected groups of children and adolescents who had to deal with the loss as well. Consider the following statistics provided by the Boston Public Schools in 1982 (the latest year for which complete figures are available at the time of writing). Fifty-two children aged three to eighteen died in Boston. Nineteen of the children were three to twelve years of age and thirty-three were aged thirteen to eighteen years. If each child in the younger group was in a preschool or elementary school class of twenty-five students, and if the death of each of the thirty-three older children affected one hundred and fifty of their peers in junior and senior high school, then those fifty-two deaths confronted a minimum of 5,424 young people with an experience of loss. These figures apply only to Boston (not the suburbs) and do not include the deaths of adults who were significant figures in the lives of groups of children.

Communities have developed good mental-health services to help bereaved family members. There are mental-health professionals in schools to help young people who develop symptoms as a result of the death of a loved one. There are few programs, however, to help groups of children deal with the death of a friend—a classmate, teacher, counselor, cook, custodian, cabin-mate at camp, or someone else who is important to them. Efforts to help groups of bereaved youngsters have usually been provided by individual principals, guidance counselors, school nurses, or camp directors or by persons in a community mental-health program serving a particular catchment area. There has been little opportunity, therefore, to build a body of experience or to develop a conceptual or service-delivery model for responding to such situations.

CRISIS AND PREVENTION

The death of a friend is a serious challenge to the coping skills of children and adolescents. Early intervention by adults who are a part of their everyday lives makes it possible to keep these young people psychologically healthy and to prevent the development of later emotional problems. Primary prevention programs use a public-health model, providing services to all members of a vulnerable population. Interventions are oriented to stressful life events. The traditional emphasis on the treatment of troubled children and families is replaced by the promotion of health and the prevention of disease. The most effective prevention activities are based in institutions that are a part of the community's daily life—schools, churches, and work sites, for example. As Okin (1977:296) stated, "The school system—with its captive audience, its tendency to induce strong transferential ties between teachers and students, and the very central place it occupies in the life of the child and the community—is an ideal institution for promoting health and preventing disability."

Cowen (1983:15) identified primary prevention programs. These programs must be:

(1) Mass-oriented or group-oriented, not targeted to individuals;
(2) Directed to essentially well people, not to those who are already affected, though targets can appropriately include those who, by virtue of life

circumstances or recent experiences, are known (epidemiologically) to be at risk for adverse psychological outcomes;

(3) "Intentional"; that is, rest on a knowledge base that suggests that a program's operations hold promise for strengthening psychological health or reducing psychological maladjustment.

The death of a friend, as stated earlier, is a significant and stressful event in the lives of groups of children and adolescents. Most adults clearly remember from childhood their friends or teachers who died. Many remember equally clearly that no one discussed those deaths with them. There is now a great deal of evidence, however, to support the value of helping groups of bereaved children deal with the death of a friend. We know that the death of someone who is an important part of their lives leaves young people vulnerable and at risk for physical, emotional, and behavioral problems. Osterweis, Solomon, and Green's (1984) report to the Institute of Medicine discussed these issues in detail. We also know that it is possible to "immunize" or "inoculate" young people psychologically by helping them to deal with less intense losses so that they will not be overwhelmed by later, more personally meaningful deaths (Kliman 1968; Zusman 1975). Gordon and Klass (1979:90) wrote that "students who have been members of a school community that handled death well will be able to cope with death in the various communities they join as adults." Finally, we know that the pathological sequelae of unhealthy coping with bereavement can be prevented if community caretakers help people mourn adequately (Lindemann 1944, 1979).

TASKS FOR GROUPS OF BEREAVED CHILDREN AND ADOLESCENTS

When a friend dies, groups of children or adolescents lose someone who has been a part of their lives and activities. Since the normal and predictable response to loss is grief, the concern is not whether the youngsters will grieve, but whether their grief will be healthy or pathological. Adults can play an important role in assuring that the grief is *good* grief — that it helps the surviving group of youngsters stay psychologically healthy and that it strengthens their capacity to cope with future losses. To grieve successfully, groups of bereaved children and adolescents must accomplish four tasks:

Understanding This task involves knowing that the person is no longer alive — that his or her body has stopped working — and that the person will never again be part of the group in the same way. Completion of this task requires the provision of honest age-appropriate information that dispels rumors.

Grieving The children must experience and express the feelings that go with the loss, including sadness, anger, and guilt. The specific content of the grief will depend on the children's relationship with the person who died, on the cause of death, and on a variety of other factors.

Commemorating This is the process of formally or informally remembering the life (rather than the death) of the person who died. The friends of the one who died need to be involved in the final decisions about how their friend will be remembered. Commemoration confirms both the reality of the death and the value of human life.

Going On After they complete the first three tasks, groups of children need to resume their usual activities of living, learning, and loving. Brown (1958) described this task in her classic children's book, *The Dead Bird,* when she spoke about how, in time, the children forgot their daily ritual of putting flowers on their bird's grave and singing to the bird. It is not quite accurate to say that children "forget." Having dealt with the death and with the grief, they can go on with living.

THE GOOD GRIEF PROGRAM

The ideas and challenges described in this article have been drawn from the author's experience as founder and director of the Good Grief Program in Boston, Massachusetts. The Good Grief Program is a primary prevention program, co-sponsored by the Judge Baker Guidance Center and the Junior League of Boston. The goal of the Good Grief Program is to help schools and community groups become a base of support for children and adolescents when a friend dies. The administration of the program and all clinical services are handled by the program director, who is a member of the staff at Judge Baker Guidance Center, a child mental-health agency. Approximately fifteen volunteers, coordinated by the Junior League, help with outreach, lead discussion groups as part of Good Grief's educational programs, and prepare resource materials. Fees for the services are billed at an hourly rate. Schools and community groups are expected to meet the cost of services to the greatest extent possible. We believe that it is essential for their budgets to include funds for preventive mental-health services and we work with groups to achieve this goal. The program receives important community sanction and financial support from foundations, corporations, and individual contributors.

The Good Grief Program offers five services: crisis intervention, consultation, in-service training, educational programs, and the development and provision of resource materials.

Crisis Intervention

The staff meet with groups of children or adolescents to talk about the terminal illness or recent death of a friend. Adults from the school or community group are present so that they can continue to be available to the youngsters over time. The following is an example of this service.

> The day after eleven-year-old Betsy was raped and murdered in a neighborhood park, staff from the community center where she was a member

of the Girls' Club asked the director of the Good Grief Program to meet with Betsy's fellow club members. The Girls' Club leader, overwhelmed by her own feelings about Betsy's brutal death, could only sob and tell the club members how much she loved them. With her permission, however, the girls were able to ask the director of the Good Grief Program many questions about their own safety, why anyone would want to hurt young girls, what to expect at the wake and funeral, the trouble they were having eating and sleeping, and the multitude of other things that were worrying them.

Consultation

The staff meet with an individual or a small group of school administrators, program staff, teachers, or others who, after discussion and planning, are then able to respond to the needs of a group of children or adolescents, as can be seen in this example:

Late one evening, the superintendent of a rural school system called with the following story. At noon that day, a five-year-old girl got off the kindergarten bus, headed up the walk toward her house, and suddenly dashed back to pick up something she had dropped under the bus. The driver did not see her and drove on. The child's fatal injuries were observed not only by her mother and the bus driver, but by the fifteen kindergarten students who were still on the bus. The superintendent sought consultation on the following issues: contacting the parents of the child who had died; responding to the mental-health needs of the bus driver; emotionally supporting the siblings of the child who had died and the children of the bus driver; anticipating the predictable needs of the surviving classmates and other students in the school; commemorating the life of the dead child, who had just entered the school four weeks earlier and was not yet well known by anyone; helping the kindergarten teacher, who had stayed home on the day of the accident; and dealing with parents who were concerned about the safety of children riding on the school bus. Within an hour, which was all the time that was available then, a plan was developed to address these issues; roles and responsibilities were also defined.

In-Service Training

Seminars or workshops are designed and conducted for the faculty of a school, a group of nurses, the guidance staff of a school system, camp directors, or others who are responsible for groups of children or adolescents and who may be called on to help them deal with the death of a friend, as in the following instance:

After hearing about the Good Grief Program, the director of the guidance department of a large suburban high school invited the director of the Good Grief Program to address the school's monthly faculty meeting. The presentation, "Helping Groups of Adolescents Deal with Death and Dying," was followed by two after-school workshops for interested teachers and counselors. Approximately fifteen people met to talk about ways to include discussions of death and dying in the school's existing curriculum, about handling the death of a recent graduate who had not been an outstanding member of the school community, and about students whose schoolwork had deteriorated after the death of a family member.

Education Programs

Presentations are made to parent-teacher organizations, church groups, and other community groups who are interested in ways to help children deal with a particular death or with the general topic of death and dying. These educational programs are not necessarily given during a crisis, but they are also appropriate at the time a death occurs, as in the example that follows:

> Jim's collapse and unexpected death on the school playground shocked and stunned his fourth-grade classmates, who were there when it happened, and their parents. Now, two months later, the parents still had many questions of their own and were finding that their children did, too. At an evening PTA-sponsored meeting, a staff member from the Good Grief Program shared what is known about children and death and showed the videotaped puppet program, "The Death of a Friend: Helping Children Cope with Grief and Loss." Parents and teachers then met in small discussion groups led by volunteers of the program. The evening offered a variety of opportunities for discussion and made clear to all that parents, children, and teachers were still scared and suffering. The most pressing questions were what the still-unexplained cause of death meant about the vulnerability of all children, and uncertainties about whether the children had understood the efforts by school personnel to resuscitate Jim or else had interpreted them as being the thing that had actually killed him.
>
> Following this evening of discussion, the parents of all fourth graders decided to meet with the teachers and other school personnel to view the videotape again and to discuss ongoing ways to support this frightened group of youngsters.

Resource Materials

The staff and volunteers of the Good Grief Program have developed the following resource materials:

- *The Death of a Friend: Helping Children Cope with Grief and Loss.* A puppet presentation (available in video and film formats) featuring Susan Linn. Available for sale or rent from New Dimension Films, 85895 Lorane Highway, Eugene, Oregon 97405.
- *Good Grief: Helping Groups of Children When a Friend Dies.* A book about the design and services of the Good Grief Program in Boston. Available from the Good Grief Program.
- *An Annotated Bibliography of Books and Films for Children and Adolescents About Death and Dying.* An annotated listing of books and films indicating who died, the cause of death, racial or ethnic focus, whether the setting is urban, suburban, or rural, reading level, and strengths or limitations. Available from the Good Grief Program.

- *Death Education Resources and Materials for Preschools and Elementary and Secondary Schools: An Annotated Guide.* A description of books, articles, and curricula to assist those who are developing or offering death education programs. Available from the Good Grief Program.
- *Cultural and Ethnic Rituals and Observances at the Time of Death.* Information for teachers and others who work with groups of children about the usual rituals and observances of many ethnic and cultural groups in America today. Available from the Good Grief Program.

RESEARCH ON STRESSFUL LIFE EVENTS

The outcomes of preventive intervention programs are of great interest to those who design and deliver mental health services. Bloom (1985:1) wrote that the "identification of stressful life events (contemporary or recent external events that make adaptive demands on a person) in a community, combined with the development of appropriate intervention programs, may be one of the keys to the effective prevention of much emotional distress." Research on prevention, however, poses unusually complex methodological problems, particularly when the stressful life event to be studied involves children. There is unanimous agreement on the need for prospective studies, and strong encouragement for the use of the cohort control method (contrasting a group of children who have experienced a particular event with a matched group of youngsters who have not) in order to determine whether a suspected outcome has occurred significantly more often in the group of children who have experienced the event.

Particular challenges arise in designing research to study the impact of the death of a friend on a group of children and to determine the outcomes that can be attributed to intervention, such as that offered by the Good Grief Program. To do prospective studies and to begin to collect data in a timely fashion, it would be best to obtain informed consent from parents and schools as soon as possible after the death of a friend of a group of children. However, as was true in the early days of sex education in the schools, many parents, school personnel, and community groups are not convinced that children should talk about the death of a friend when it occurs. Many adults who could help children deal with loss and grief do not feel adequately prepared for the task and hesitate to proceed for fear they will say or do the wrong thing. Furthermore, the strong commitment to treatment rather than to prevention results in the development of services for those who do not cope well and become symptomatic, not for all who have been exposed to a particular stressful life event.

Before one can expect to gain access to the children to be studied, therefore, in-service training and educational programs will be needed to create opportunities to talk with adults about the importance of preventive intervention programs as a resource for promoting the future mental health of young people. The Good Grief Program considers that its current services of education and training for adults and the development of relationships with schools and community groups are the first step in the process of studying the impact of the death of a friend on groups of children, and in determining what kind of services have favorable outcomes with which youngsters in what kinds of situations.

The program has begun to ask schools and community groups to share their thoughts about the services they have used. Each of the thirty-two responses has noted that the program had been "very helpful." These responses have come from eighteen public schools, six preschools, one private school, one special-needs day school, one residential program for handicapped youngsters, one church, one patient-activity program in a hospital, one hospice, one parochial school, and one area health agency. Services were provided to eleven of those schools and community organizations at a time of crisis; there was no specific situation that precipitated the calls from the other twenty-one, but many were dissatisfied with their handling of a recent death with a group of children.

The groups described the following as the "most important thing" they had learned from the Good Grief Program:

- The appropriate things to say or do with classes when there has been a death or loss.
- Not to play down or ignore the emotions unleashed by tragedies.
- That children are aware of death and can be helped to understand and cope positively with death and dying; that adults' discomfort and lack of information are no longer acceptable reasons for excluding children from rituals or discussions of death.
- As staff, we should acknowledge our own feelings about loss as we try to help children and their families deal with theirs.

Others mentioned the importance of information about the development of children's understanding of death; being available, aware, and willing to listen; the ways in which children express grief; the provision of concrete information to dispel rumors; and children's need to learn about death and dying on an ongoing basis rather than just at time of crisis.

We also asked schools and community groups what they had done differently since the Good Grief Program had worked with them. Again, the responses varied, often in relation to the particular need that had precipitated the request for services.

- The representative of a high school that had dealt with a student's suicide wrote: "We speak of suicide more openly, encouraging students to suggest alternatives to situations in the literature. Hotline phone numbers are prominently displayed. I have had individual conferences with grieving or at-risk students to offer services or sympathy. The shuttle disaster occurred during school time. Many of us felt more confident about helping the students respond to the tragedy. In teaching Romeo and Juliet, I point out Friar Lawrence's speech to Romeo as a fine example of counseling a person who is suicidal."

- A school nurse in an inner-city elementary school said, "I recognized the types of behavior that are manifestations of grief. All students with behavioral problems are now routinely referred to me."
- A health educator in a school system that used the Good Grief Program the day after two high school students were killed in an automobile accident noted, "We dealt more directly with the questions that the children had about the space shuttle disaster. We talked about the dangerous move a New Hampshire principal made by taking students out of the viewing room where they were watching television when the disaster happened."
- A school system that was troubled by a number of student, parent, and faculty deaths, wrote, "Plans are underway to put together a committee to address the development of a plan or strategy for handling a tragedy."
- A special-needs teacher who asked for crisis intervention for her students following the unexpected death of a nineteen-year-old with muscular dystrophy (one of three in the class with that illness) reported: "We seem to be talking more openly and sharing our feelings, especially about the young man who died. We can talk about him and feel good about it."
- The psychologist in an elementary school that had to deal with the suicide of its principal said: "I am much more sensitive to death and grieving and now incorporate discussions of death in my classroom units. It is gradually becoming part of the curriculum. All elementary schools now have books on death in their libraries and the librarians read and discuss these stories with the children."

Others commented on the development of adolescent-suicide support services; on planned meeting times to discuss issues of loss that affect staff, children, and families; and on their increased confidence in their ability to help students cope with grief and loss. Several schools noted the need for another presentation to address a larger staff group than was initially served. A number of the schools and community groups that initially requested consultation or small in-service training activities are now scheduling educational programs for parents and for larger groups of their own staff, and are telling others about the importance of using resources like the Good Grief Program.

During the first year of its activity (1983-84), the Good Grief Program received ninety-six inquiries or requests for service, mostly from metropolitan Boston, and provided direct services to forty-nine schools or community groups, teaching 2,080 persons through those services. In 1984-85, the program received 430 inquiries or requests for service and provided direct services to seventy-four schools or community groups, reaching 3,139 persons through those services. During the first half of 1985-86, the program received 387 inquiries or requests for service from all over the United States and from eight foreign countries, provided direct services in forty-five situations (with thirty-five scheduled for the second half of the year), and reached 2,909 persons. I believe that community interest in preventive services for groups of children when a friend dies has been well documented. The program makes good sense to schools and community groups. It must now also direct its efforts toward a clearer understanding of what works best and why.

REFERENCES

Bloom, B. L. 1985. *Stressful Life Event Theory and Research: Implications for Primary Prevention.* Rockville MD: National Institute of Mental Health.

Brown, M. W. 1958. *The Dead Bird.* Reading MA: Addison-Wesley.

Cowen, E. L. 1983. "Primary Prevention in Mental Health: Past, Present, and Future." In R. D. Felner et al., eds. *Preventive Psychology: Theory, Research, and Practice.* New York: Pergamon Press.

Gordon, A. K. and D. Klass. 1979. *They Need to Know: How to Teach Children About Death.* Englewood Cliffs NJ: Prentice-Hall.

Kliman, G. 1968. *Psychological Emergencies of Childhood.* New York: Grune & Stratton.

Lindemann, E. 1944. "Symptomatology and Management of Acute Grief." *American Journal of Psychiatry* 101:141–148.

Lindemann, E. 1979. *Beyond Grief: Studies in Crisis Intervention.* New York: Jason Aronson.

Okin, R. L. 1977. "Primary Prevention of Psychopathology from the Perspective of a State Mental Health Program Director." In G. W. Albee and J. M. Jaffee, eds. *Primary Prevention of Psychopathology,* vol. 1: Hanover NH: University Press of New England.

Osterweis, M., F. Solomon, and M. Green, eds. 1984. *Bereavement: Reactions, Consequences, and Care.* Washington DC: National Academy Press.

Zusman, J. 1975. "Primary Prevention." In A. M. Freedman, H. I. Kaplan, and B. J. Sadock, eds. *Comprehensive Textbook of Psychiatry.* II. Baltimore MD: Williams & Wilkins.

9

Prevention in Major Childhood Bereavement:

A Psychosocial View

Stephen Lubowe

This chapter is an adaptation to major childhood bereavements of Cassel's theory of the nature of suffering and its prevention or amelioration. Major bereavements are roughly synonymous with the major psychological emergencies of childhood according to Kliman (1968): illness and death in the family; divorce; and adoption. Cassel (1982) proposed a simplified typology of the whole person that can be used to investigate and prevent or ameliorate suffering; to wit, three dimensions of personhood — the personal, the social, and the transcendent. Suffering happens when "...the impending destruction of the person is perceived, it continues until the threat of disintegration has passed or until the integrity of the person can be resumed in some other manner" (Cassel 1982:640). There is the concept of resilience in which recovery from suffering (the loss of parts of one's life) is possible; there may even be a different level of integration in the expression of the dimensions of one's personhood. An examination of the cause of suffering in the personal, social, and transcendent dimension is, therefore, warranted.

CAUSES OF SUFFERING IN THE PERSONAL DIMENSION

Attachment is the emotional bond of affective energy that is invested in any important object. Disattachment, grief, or bereavement may be defined as the stressful, painful psychological reaction that is put in motion by an anticipated or actual break in the emotional bond — a response to loss of the affective tie or injury to one's personal integrity. Disattachment results in "Many forms of emotional distress and personality disturbance, including anxiety, anger, depression, and emotional detachment" arising from involuntary separation and loss (Bowlby 1980:39). An example of this profound influence is the statistical correlation between a death in the family in early childhood and "later-life learning disabilities, school failures, juvenile delinquency, and adult-life hospitalization for depressive illness" (Kliman and Rosenfeld 1980:261).

Stages of Loss

One can anlayze the following five typical stages of object loss at different ages and including individual differences (Grollman 1967; Kübler-Ross 1969; Nieburg and Fischer 1982).

Denial This is a natural defense reaction against the reality of death that gives one a chance to mobilize one's psychological resources and regain one's equilibrium (Kübler-Ross 1969, Nieburg and Fischer 1982). Immediately after the emotional trauma (pathogenic experience) of receiving the shocking news (the diagnosis or the notification of death), most children react with numbed disbelief because the loss seems unreal. A major theme of Kliman's work is how parents' denial and avoidance of sharing the painful truth of a loss, such as the death of a pet, because of a mistaken desire to shield children from short-term discomfort, leave children more vulnerable to long-term suffering and damaging psychopathology. The denial of death and the "defensive noncommunication" of the tragic realities of life are, to some extent, a product of the attitudes of contemporary American society toward illness and death and children (Kliman 1968, Kliman and Rosenfeld 1980).

Anger When denial wears off, one may feel angry at the loss of the loved one (Feinberg 1970, Grollman 1967, Kübler-Ross 1969, Nieburg and Fischer 1982). The child's anger at being abandoned by the beloved one who became ill or died is increased when the child is denied complete participation in the remaining family activities. The other children may be angry when a dying sibling monopolizes their parents' time. As the bearer of bad news, the physician may be the scapegoat for irrational anger. The bereaved person's hostility (both a reaction to abandonment and a plea for attention) is a source of resistance to referral and or treatment (Kliman 1968).

Guilt The next stage is blaming oneself, or guilt (Grollman 1967, Kliman 1968, Kliman and Rosenfeld 1980, Nieburg and Fischer 1982). Those who are bereaved often feel irrational, unreasonable guilt about their neglect of or harmful behavior toward the lost person. The psychoanalytic tradition emphasizes excessive ambivalence (combining feelings of love and hate) and the attendant guilt as important factors in self-punitive identification with the lost person and as problems in the resolution of grief. Children often feel guilty because of their omnipotent, magical thinking; that is, they may have wished that the loved one would go away or die and they may irrationally consider the responsibility for the separation, increased illness, or death to be a punishment.

Depression and anxiety These are other important, painful feelings (Kliman 1968, Nieburg and Fischer 1982). For bereaved persons, depression often accompanies guilt, since both feelings stem from low self-evaluation and the need for self-reproach and chastisement because of their inability to save the loved one. Depression may take days or months to pass, and may prevent the bereaved person from living a normal life. It may involve such physical symptoms as fatigue, loss of appetite, breathing and digestive dysfunctions, headaches, and sleeplessness, as well as such psychological symptoms as helplessness, apathy, ineffectiveness, and anxiety (reflected in phenomena from nightmares to lack of concentration) (Grollman 1967, Kliman 1968, Nieburg and Fischer 1982).

Anxiety can also be seen in the normal bereavement reactions of "pangs" of grief or separation anxiety (Parkes 1975). When bereaved persons experience grief pangs, they pine over the absent loved one and have episodes of extreme anxiety that often are highlighted by involuntary weeping. These spontaneous reactions begin within hours or days of bereavement (the post-denial period) and gradually decrease in frequency. The grief episodes also include hyperactivity, preoccupation with memories of the deceased (such as "bereavement hallucinations"), and inability to concentrate on the ordinary pleasurable aspects of life. The bereavement symptoms may be part of the urge to recover the lost person.

Acceptance When one has worked through denial, anger, guilt, depression, and anxiety, one can reach the acceptance stage and resume ordinary life. Because the time it takes to work through bereavement varies from person to person, family conflicts can arise—for example, when a newly widowed parent sees his or her adolescent going to play sports just after the other parent's death (Kliman 1968, Nieburg and Fischer 1982).

Two tasks of the bereavement period can go awry. First, the bereaved must accept the reality of death and the end of the relationship with the deceased. The lack of a funeral ritual can hinder this acceptance, particularly with children. Preventing children from participating in the funeral and seeing the deceased's body, if they wish to do so, can stimulate their fantasies. It is best to deal forthrightly with the painful feelings engendered by a loss (Grollman 1957, Kliman 1968). Second, parents who deny or avoid sharing the harsh truth of a loss with children may help create later problems; they may miss the opportunity to strengthen the children psychologically through the immunizing value of communicating truths. The parent may either unwisely omit an explanation for the loss of a pet or of a parent (from death or divorce) or answer the child's questions with euphemisms. These types of responses can cause the child to lose confidence in the parent during the bereavement period (Grollman 1967, Kliman 1968). Dealing with the pain of the loss may be harder when there is no sympathetic social network to share it, to help with the everyday routine, to offer spiritual and psychological support, and to contribute to a sense of continuity during the stressful period.

Obstacles to Bereavement

The resolution of bereavement means that the bereaved has accepted the finality of death, worked through and decathected memories of the lost object so that they have become more pleasurable than painful, and formed new relations. Children, for example, seek new substitute object relations after the death of a parent (Grollman 1967; Kliman 1968). Two major obstacles to the recovery of whole personhood are abnormal bereavement and fear of bereavement.

Abnormal bereavement This is intense and extended grief when there is unmitigated, indefinite bereavement and nonacceptance of object loss (Kliman 1968, Lindemann 1975, Nieburg and Fischer 1982). The person has had a special or complex relationship to the lost object, such as a relationship that involved extreme ambivalence. Kliman's (1968) prospective study of eighteen untreated orphans showed that the age of children and the mental health of their parents are important in predicting psychological illness in children. The key factors were extreme youth: for girls, the death of the mother before the girls reach eight years; and for boys, the death of the father during the boys' adolescence. A parent's mental illness and a poor relationship between the child and either the dead or the remaining parent are significant, but the sudden suicide of a mentally ill parent is especially predictive of abnormal bereavement in children.

Fear of bereavement People who are too frightened to grieve are overwhelmed by a chaotic, unnerving flood of various feelings (such as helplessness) and symptoms (including uncontrollable insomnia). Deutsch (1975) was the first to speak of the "absence of grief" associated with the loss of a parent. When an individual does not manifestly grieve immediately, the pain of grief is not permanently suppressed, but shows up in later years ("double mourning").

CAUSES OF SUFFERING IN THE SOCIAL DIMENSION

The causes of suffering in the personal dimension extend from family, school, and health-care professionals to include the broader areas of societal institutions and cultural expectations.

The Family

Within families, suffering can be induced by the less-than-optimal management of the intellectual and affective issues of object loss. When information about a psychological crisis is withheld from children or transmitted in a way that is evasive or incomprehensible (for example, if it is expressed at an inappropriate cognitive level), psychological dysfunction can result. In the emotional area, parents or parental figures may fail to provide a successful, directive model of grief management by honest expression and communication. Parents may fail to use or may improperly use specific techniques to facilitate healthy bereavement; for example, they may not encourage children to participate actively in planning and carrying out their preferences for the funeral and burial.

The School

This environment may not be used properly to reduce or prevent suffering in childhood's major bereavements through the application of psychological immunization techniques and a liaison approach to children with life-threatening illnesses. The power of synergistic interaction among the school, the family, and health care professionals may be ignored, as may the use of research while providing education services.

Psychological immunization Opportunities may not be taken for psychological strengthening (prevention) through immunizing discussions with preschoolers of everyday tragedies like the loss of a pet (Kliman 1968, Nieburg and Fischer 1982) or with older children of national psychological crises, such as the assassination of President John Kennedy (Kliman 1968, Liman and Rosenfeld 1989). School administrators and teachers may decide to shield children or to delay the communication of the tragic news. Crisis communications may not be managed in the best manner. For example, the teacher may fail as a role model in expressing uncontrolled or inappropriate emotions; and there may be no opportunity for the children to participate in a full, organized, supportive classroom discussion. By not using the classroom for psychological immunization, the schools neglect a way of facilitating communication at home between parents and children about life's crises.

Liaison approach The absence or poor management of a school liaison program for children with life-threatening illnesses may induce suffering (Deasy-Spinetta and Spinetta 1983). Children who are not told the full truth about the illness and who are not allowed to discuss it forthrightly are prevented from functioning optimally in all areas, including school. Teachers who are ignorant of a child's disease, or who do not have a viable philosophy and mature emotional perspective regarding death cannot provide a nurturing and supportive environment. A teacher who is ill-prepared does not have a knowledgeable interest in the normal psychological and developmental needs of the dying student, or an awareness of the importance of family dynamics. An inadequate school liaison approach mismanages the child's reentry into school by neglecting class discussions; mishandles school referral by failing to identify problems; and neglects the education of teachers by failing to conduct interdisciplinary seminars.

The Society

The state of our social institutions and the lack of sufficient government funds for high-quality child care and related programs are symptomatic of the national neglect of children's priority in our "child-centered" society. Specifically, this neglect can be seen in the lack of preventive programs for many important problems related to children's physical and mental health: infant mortality, inadequate nutrition and shelter, hyperactivity, and child abuse. As yet there is no cohesive, flexibly implemented social policy concerned with the welfare of children in the United States. An optimal program would not ignore the psychological importance of the early attachment of parent and child and the need for responsible involvement in humanized social institutions.

The breakdown of the extended family and the old support systems is part of the oft-noted rise of alienation in all social institutions and spheres of contemporary American society. This alienation can be seen in two important interrelated areas that are relevant to childhood's major bereavements: educational and social situations, and preventive mental health services.

Education and social situations The non-localized child care system of traditional life has been replaced by the nuclear family guided by professional experts. The family neighborhood is no longer the primary socializer; this function is increasingly provided by the "antisocial" peer group and the mass media (Brofenbrenner 1973). The maintenance of this situation depends on the contribution of numerous alienating conditions: inadequate day care, poor job rewards, and inflexible work schedules; the segregation of children from adults with the lack of joint participation in work; the secondary role of American women; the denial of the child's need for important responsibilities; poor neighborhood and urban planning; and inadequate adoption and child placement procedures.

Mental health services Contemporary American mental health services neglect the importance of prevention, particularly for preschoolers. Our society may be in danger of a mass psychological "epidemic" of preschoolers who are at risk for a lifetime of emotional illness (Kliman and Rosenfeld 1980, Rosenfeld 1976). By the time they reach school age, it may be too late to give these children significant help; enormous amounts of time and money may be required for rescue efforts that may only partially arrest the damage.

Preventive mental health services for children are inadequate for several reasons:

1. Established practices mandate that about 70 percent of all mental health money be spent on the institutionalization of severely ill poor adults and the confused elderly; this seemingly unbalanced priority exacts a great cost both financially and emotionally.
2. Community mental health centers — the alternative to institutionalization — receive about 4 percent of the national mental health budget, virtually none of which is used for preventive and children's mental health services (Albee 1985, Kliman and Rosenfeld 1980).
3. Prevailing cultural attitudes about mental health and the prevention of mental illness in young children foster public unconcern about the danger of a mass psychological disaster and inadequate mental health services. The public has been neither educated nor involved in constructive solutions (Albee 1984, Kliman and Rosenfeld 1980).
4. There is a belief in traditional health care circles that "alternative" preventive treatment (stressing health and the avoidance of illness over the treatment of disease and illness) is not essential and lacks scientific validation. The subsection of the National Institute of Mental Health that deals with prevention has not received sufficient governmental backing (Albee 1985, Gelman et al. 1985, McPheeters 1977).
5. Community mental health centers have emphasized the diagnostic evaluation of children over treatment, and there is no national effort to provide more trained child therapists in this emotionally demanding and arduous profession (Kliman and Rosenfeld 1980, McPheeters 1977).

Cultural Attitudes

Suffering is induced in childhood's major bereavements by interrelated cultural attitudes about the "low priority" areas of children, bereavement, and preventive health care. This society has a self-fulfilling negative view of children's psychological stamina and ability to handle responsibility which is interconnected with the view that children should be shielded from life's harsh realities. The result is that children often are not allowed to participate in family decisions about object loss, such as illness and death in the family. In addition, children with life-threatening illnesses are often not treated like dignified individuals who are entitled to honest communication with the family and the health care team (Kliman 1968, Parkes 1983).

For severely ill children and their families, suffering is sometimes induced by the modern hospital's emphasis on physical needs to the exclusion of psychosocial ones, and on cure and survival over quality of life and overall emotional well-being (Cassel 1975, Kübler-Ross 1969). The policies and practices of many hospitals do little to counter alienation and stressful, negative feelings. For the young child with a life-threatening illness, the important stabilizing routine of family contact is interrupted. The fear of death and the stress of painful hospital procedures such as chemotherapy and radiation may not have been mitigated by preparatory, immunizing discussions about illness and hospitalization. The hospital milieu may actually hinder open communication among the child, the family, and the health care team. These factors contribute to the child's feelings of isolation, helplessness, anger, anxiety, guilt, and sadness. Family members may experience similar feelings as they try to work through their bereavement and to support each other. Parents may find it hard to communicate forthrightly with the child about important issues such as radiation therapy and possible disfigurement, and may not pay sufficient attention to their other children or provide them with reassurance.

The hospital team is subject to the same stressful emotions, including loneliness, insecurity, and hostility, and there may be interstaff conflict. The hospital team may be inattentive in supporting the family; for example, after the child has died the team may make the mistake of not attending the funeral and sending condolences (Marten and Mauer 1983; Solnit 1983).

On the other hand, the prevalent model of health care may overemphasize the importance of professionals and the treatment of illness and underemphasize the importance of nonprofessionals who are involved in voluntary associations, holistic self-help care, and the prevention of illness. The new humanistic model of health care stresses a more balanced and symmetrical view of responsibility in a larger health care framework that includes prevention. Health care cannot be optimal without cooperation among the health care team, the child, and the family with regard to active decision making, without peer therapy and support groups for parents and children, and without interdisciplinary staff meetings for professionals to help prevent emotional disorders (Binger et al. 1983, Haslack 1982, Solnit 1983).

CAUSES OF SUFFERING IN THE TRANSCENDENT DIMENSION

In this dimension, there are two causes of suffering: the loss of values and the absence of "community." In childhood's major bereavements, the appearance of a life crisis or psychological emergency can shake up the values of children and families as they seek to cope with it. Our cultural perspective about children, bereavement, and preventive care, as well as sociopolitical obstacles, have hindered children, families, and professionals from gaining a sense of secular transcendence as a community working toward the ideals of equality, self-determination, and human dignity (Bensman and Rosenberg 1976, Cassel 1982).

PREVENTION OR AMELIORATION OF SUFFERING IN THE PERSONAL DIMENSION

By adapting Liebow's (1967) view of simultaneous intervention at all points in the problems, we can use Cassel's (1975, 1982) topological analysis of personhood and suffering to develop an optimal strategy for the prevention and alleviation of suffering in childhood's major bereavements. Reducing and preventing suffering in the personal dimension (shading into the social dimension) can be analyzed by stressing a) the types of problems found and the help required (both professional and self-help), and b) psychological immunization for childhood's major psychological emergencies.

Types of Help

Professional help Professional counseling is required when one cannot spontaneously recover from a loss. Such counseling can teach the client, the family, and peers "non-defensive" communication and allow relatives and friends to provide the emotional support individuals need in order to work through the five stages of bereavement and, in so doing, to recover the lost parts of themselves and be healed.

Therapy can help individuals who are undergoing abnormal bereavement to express blocked feelings, thereby promoting recovery. In therapy, clients often are able to remember countless minute bits of experience surrounding the beloved lost object; learn to differentiate and experience a wide range of emotions, including sadness, anger, and guilt; and realistically assess the loss. Particularly when dealing with young children, the counselor may a) discuss the death of pets and distant family members in order to allow for the release of emotion; b) question the child to encourage a realistic view of the permanence of the object loss and correct any cognitive misconceptions about illness and death; and c) clarify memory images in order to aid in future bereavement (Feinberg 1970, Kliman 1968, Nieburg and Fischer 1982).

Self-help Family autoanalysis, which may involve other than the immediate family, has goals similar to those of professional help. The parents or parental figures function as "preventive psychiatrists" or "collaborating guides"; they facilitate bereavement by stressing the realistic acceptance of the loss and by dealing directly and sensitively with the feelings engendered by the loss (Grollman 1967, Kliman 1968, Kliman and Rosenfeld 1980, Nieburg and Fischer 1982). The family members seek to stimulate the detailed remembrance of events, whether pleasant or not, and to share old memories. Visiting a familiar spot or looking at old photograph albums and home movies can serve as the basis for the free expression of emotions, including negative ones, about the lost object. Written recollections are valuable, particularly for children, for bringing out hidden thoughts and feelings, which then can be more easily managed. The family's emotional health is also greatly aided by a supportive social network of relatives, friends, neighbors, professional acquaintances, and community organizations (such as Parents Without Partners, and Big Brothers). The existing social support system should be enlisted as soon as possible to provide emotional nourishment and aid in household chores (Kliman and Rosenfeld 1980, Nieburg and Fischer 1982).

Psychological Immunization

Kliman's concept of psychological immunization or mental preparedness refers to the immunizing value of the concerned adult's sharing of small doses of life's painful truths (such as thoughts and feelings about death) with the child. This important therapeutic concept for preventing and managing childhood's major bereavements across all three dimensions of personhood is based on a biomedical analogy. Physiological immunization allows the host to deal with a noxious agent without becoming very ill. Thus, a safe dose of a toxin or bacterial culture may allow immunity, whereas a large dose of the same substance given abruptly might create overwhelming illness, and a dose that might be immunizing for the adult might be dangerous for a child. In preventive psychiatry and allied disciplines, children might be exposed in a safe, controlled manner to an age-appropriate dose of anxiety in a potentially pathogenic experience; the child would develop some immunity and would be better prepared for life's inevitable crises. The immunizing concept implies that the optimal stimulating environment is neither overprotective nor underprotective.

Finally, Kliman referred to two theoretical concepts related to psychological immunization — "readiness" and "mastery in advance." Defensive excitation of the mental apparatus into intellectual and emotional readiness when faced with danger is the prototype of psychological immunization. Mastery in advance includes active dealing with stress before an event through reflective thought, fantasy rehearsal, and actual experience with weak doses of stress. Thus, mastery in advance involves small doses of anxious discomfort that can help preschoolers lessen the emotional impact of life's major bereavements (Kliman 1968, Kliman and Rosenfeld 1980).

PREVENTION OR AMELIORATION OF SUFFERING IN THE SOCIAL DIMENSION

The prevention or reduction of social suffering extends outward from the family, the school, and health care professionals to include the broader areas of cultural attitudes and social institutions. It can be seen in the optimal management of the cognitive and emotional aspects of object loss.

The Family

In psychological emergencies, from divorce to life-threatening illness and death in the family, the facts should be fully and straightforwardly explained to the child in an age-appropriate manner, as close to the time of the loss as possible. Parents should use familiar, comprehensible language; the complexity of the explanation should be consonant with the child's level of thinking. With preschoolers, who do not view death as permanent and inevitable, emotional reassurance is more important than explanation. School-age youngsters can be told directly of the loss and the attendant circumstances. To prevent possible nightmares, however, the explanation should not introduce morbid details (Grollman 1967; Nieburg and Fischer 1982). Indeed, if parents give adequate explanations and answer children's questions, they can help prevent the child from developing emotional problems and sleep disturbances. It is especially important that parents do not use the euphemism "going to sleep" in place of "death" (Grollman 1967, Nieburg and Fischer 1982). Finally, bibliotherapy, like thanatological education in the classroom, is a valuable means of fostering children's understanding of object loss. The local librarian can recommend appropriate books to parents (Nieburg and Fischer 1982, Silverman 1984, Steinmetz Ross 1967).

Parents and teachers can reassure the child that bereavement and its honest expression (crying) is normal, not a sign of weakness (Grollman 1967, Kliman and Rosenfeld 1980, Nieburg and Fischer 1982). Adults should encourage the child to communicate painful feelings of loss, regardless of the child's fear that doing so is "silly" or "immature," and — just as importantly — regardless of the adults' desire to avoid the empathic sharing of the suffering of the dying or bereaved child.

Appropriate funerals can help children master their fears, accept the end of life, and feel calm and peaceful. Since the same principles of management of bereavement apply to primary and non-primary object losses, bereavement for a pet, with its funeral and body-disposal arrangements, can become a source of psychological immunization by providing a first experience ("dress reheasal") for the later successful management of a primary object loss (Grollman 1967, Kliman 1968, Nieburg and Fischer 1982). The funeral service helps the family to accept loss and openly express their emotional reactions in a supportive social context. It also allows the child to see the dead body or casket and the location of the grave, which helps dispel some of the mystery and fantasy that surrounds death.

The School

The importance of the school for the prevention or amelioration of suffering in major bereavements can be seen in two issues: psychological immunization in the classroom and the school liaison approach to terminally ill children. Here the child, the family, the teacher, and sometimes health care personnel act in tandem to reinforce each others' efforts.

Psychological immunization The importance of the participation of young children in classroom discussions (as a source of immunizing truth) can be seen in two cases: the death of a pet and the death of a president. Clearly these two cases vary greatly in cultural importance, but both are non-primary object losses with relatively low levels of emotional investment. When a pet dies, parents can inform the teacher of the loss; the teacher can be prepared for the development of academic and behavioral problems such as decreased concentration and increased restlessness and be able to take effective action. The teacher can, for example, integrate the loss of a pet into the classroom community by guiding group discussions and supplementing these discussions with written assignments. Classroom discussions can help create a sense of belongingness through sharing grief and working through the child's loss.

The assassination of President John F. Kennedy in 1963 created a national psychological emergency and an important opportunity for psychological immunization. The best way to handle such a crisis and to prevent emotional disturbance is by the teacher's frank announcement of the tragic news and of his or her own emotions *while continuing to function.* Catharsis is accomplished in a controlled, emotionally expressive way through such reassuring, constructive classroom activities as the discussion of presidential succession (Kliman 1968, Kliman and Rosenfeld 1980). Parents can later continue the psychological immunization process at home. Finally, therapeutic nurseries are ideal settings for immunizing discussions at an optimal age for preventive mental health work. The Cornerstone School Project in Westchester County, New York, has shown that preschoolers are psychologically strong enough to share feelings about major object losses like parental death in an organized, supportive environment and with the support of adults and peers (Kliman 1968). The findings of this project have obvious implications for older children in public schools.

School liaison and the terminally ill child A second issue concerns the role of the teacher, in cooperation with parents and health care personnel, in preventing psychosocial problems and encouraging psychosocial development in the child with a life-threatening illness. The once-common practice of socially enforced avoidance and denial serve only to produce isolation and behavior problems. It is therefore important for the physician to openly communicate the diagnosis and prognosis. All of the child's questions should be answered fully. Thereafter, the child, the family, and the health care professionals can share the psychological burden (Kliman 1968, 1969). The aware child can then live a relatively normal life organized around the school day.

Deasy-Spinetta and Spinetta (1983) have discussed a school liaison program in which the teacher works with the family and health care personnel in an active approach to total care. The prepared teacher understands the physical and sociopsychological facts about the disease, including the way family dynamics are affected by stress. It is important that the teacher see the child not only as severely ill, but as a student with normal developmental needs.

In the active preventive approach to school re-entry, health care personnel transmit medical information and give support to the school personnel. The school personnel, in turn, support the child, the family, and each other. For example, the school liaison can notify the teacher about the effects of hair loss caused by the child's medication and suggest that someone explain this to the class. With this understanding the community of students could then be better able to provide support to the child. Finally, health care personnel can conduct seminars to continue to provide school personnel with information about the child.

Social and Cultural Realms

Today's healthy children are our best guarantee that tomorrow's adults will be able to deal with increasingly complex world problems in a creative, humanistic way. To this end a program of positive social and cultural change could be based on the concept of "dialectical regression" in the context of "community formation." Dialectical regression refers to a future American society that would perhaps combine the best of traditional and modern life.

The ethos of modern scientific progress, with its emphasis on prolongation of life, elimination of disease, technologically created material abundance, and bureaucratic efficiency could well accommodate a return to traditional attitudes about natural biological processes like dying, together with renewed emphasis on humane social institutions to provide emotionally gratifying solidarity, as in the strong family (Cassel 1975, Kübler-Ross 1969). The life of children would once more involve an extended-care system with all adults active as surrogate family members to all children, as Kliman and Rosenfeld (1980:289) described:

> A lot of people who are middle-aged can remember when much of our society was like a tribal village in its embrace of children. Even if they lived in some big-city neighborhood rather than a small town or rural village, they can remember how they as children were more interactive with their parents. They were perhaps aware of many of the occupations by which adults earned their living, observing people at their stores, workshops, and wagons. Almost any passing adult felt free to take joy in children's achievements — to stop and pat a child on the head to say a word of approval, to pay a compliment — or to reprimand a misbehaving child, assuming the role of surrogate parent.

Social institutions can be reformed to embrace policies and practices that reflect the importance of parental attachment in the early years as well as the need for family and neighborhood influences on social affairs. I will examine reform in two interconnected areas: educational–social situations and preventive mental health services.

Educational–social reforms Brofenbrenner (1973) noted some educational–social reforms that allow the family and neighborhood to replace isolated peer groups and television as the major socializers — day care, increased rewards for flexible employment schedules, children's observation of work roles, improving the role of women, encouraging children in real responsibilities, and positive neighborhood and urban planning. To reverse the trend in which young children's care is delegated to child specialists, parents should play a key role in the creation and administration of day care centers and actively participate as volunteers in the implementation of the programs. Such programs cannot be limited to the day care centers but must "reach out into the home and community so the whole neighborhood is caught up in activities in behalf of children" (Brofenbrenner 1973:xvii).

Kliman and Rosenfeld (1980:288–299) noted that in this age of single-parent homes and working mothers, a large increase is needed in the number of well-trained workers ("substitute mothers") to provide high-quality day care.

- Business and governmental employers should look for ways to increase the status and pay of part-time work. Organizations should adopt policies and programs to aid family life. Parents with children in their formative years should not be penalized for spending more time at home.
- Some of the negative effects of our segregation of children from adults can be countered by allowing children to observe competent family and neighborhood adult role models at work. Organizations should encourage programs for children to visit their parents at work. Employees could "adopt" a group of children (such as a class at school) to observe and participate in their work.
- Brofenbrenner (1973:xviii) stated that in an egalitarian society, working women would get a fair deal in the home so that, in the pressured nuclear family, they could choose the most constructive child-rearing arrangement to provide optimal care.
- In this society, children are typically given unimportant, adult-supervised "rote" duties. This protection from supposedly burdensome responsibilities in fact contributes to children's incapacity to cope with difficult situations that involve real responsibilities. "Character education" could be re-introduced in functional courses of human development to encourage generativity by having older students tutor younger ones and escort them to Head Start centers.
- The neighborhood's "ecology" has a great influence on children. Jacobs (1961) analyzed the sources of successful neighborhoods, noting that in Boston, the "poor" North End had optimal material conditions and community feeling; the latter could be seen in the common concern

for children's safety in sidewalk surveillance. This neighborhood had one of the lowest crime, disease, and infant mortality rates in the state.

To this list, I will add a final reform: adoption and child placement. Some agencies have delayed the adoption of infants for months in order to provide a detailed check on children and on prospective parents. Without a single stable caretaker (mother substitute) to give high-quality care, however, emotional damage may ensue (Kliman 1968). Foster care agencies and family court judges should be guided by a flexible policy of keeping and placing children in the most optimal parental-attachment environment and of not separating abandoned siblings (Kliman and Rosenfeld 1980).

Preventive mental health centers Centers for preventive psychiatry and mental health, broadly modeled on the Westchester one, would combat the neglect of preschoolers' mental health and help foster a comprehensive view that would involve the active participation of local citizens. In the United States, hosts of preschoolers may be at high risk of a lifetime of emotional illness; thus, the earlier the psychiatric intervention, the better the chance of stopping the development of psychopathology.

The Cornerstone School of the Center for Preventive Psychiatry has found a way to counter the lack of preventive mental health services for preschoolers by maximizing the therapist's effective use of scarce time for children. The school synergistically combines the goals of child analysis with the educational process of the nursery school. The analyst works an hour and a half in the classroom and two teachers conduct classroom educational activities for three hours a day. In the familiar environment of the classroom, the interaction between classmates and teachers provides a way to accelerate insight for more than one student at a time (Kliman 1968, 1975; Rosenfeld 1976). The center also handles about 300 preschoolers a year, as well as people of all ages, in its situational crisis program (Kliman and Rosenfeld 1980, Rosenfeld 1976). The center has educated Westchester County residents to bring in their children for psychological emergencies as readily and immediately as they would for medical emergencies and has educated local child specialists, such as teachers and those in community organizations, to be on the alert for incipient problems in preschoolers and to refer them to the center for brief preventive or rescue work. As Kliman and Rosenfeld (1980:262) stated:

> We try to get adults or teenagers to act, on a long-term basis, as special friends to young, troubled children, providing someone else who cares about and who will spend significant amounts of time with them. We sought, whenever possible, and with heartwarming success, to enlist the support of people — newspaper editors, beauty parlors (sic), policemen — to act collectively as an at-the-ready network committed to whatever prompt assistance may be needed by troubled youngsters and their hard pressed young parents and families.

The center's service has rescued many preschoolers who might have not been treated by therapists or agencies in the catchment area or who might otherwise have been diagnosed as autistic or incurably retarded and spent unnecessary time in custodial care. The center has combined excellent services for the major psychological emergencies of childhood with high-quality research focused on specific variables (Kliman and Rosenfeld 1980, Rosenfeld 1976).

Children with life-threatening illnesses   Children who are dying should be in an environment, such as a home or hospice, that is more comfortable than an impersonal hospital and that is focused on enhancing the quality of the child's remaining life. In such an environment, children could receive care without being separated from parents, siblings, and other loved ones (Binger, Ablin, Kushner, and Perin 1983; Buckingham 1983; Rolsky 1983). Their mutually supportive, well-prepared family members, in conjunction with the health care team, would allow the child to die at home, but with modern medical equipment and the use of pain medication).

The home care process would permit family members, with the aid of the health care team, to work through anticipatory and subsequent bereavement together. Besides the decreased emotional cost to all concerned, the financial cost to society might well be less with home care than with hospitalization (Martinson 1983).

Finally, the medical profession and allied health disciplines should include in their programs for children and their families preventive self-help care that emphasizes the individual's whole personhood. The health care profession should institute an approach that is more egalitarian and less recipient/patient-oriented. The asymmetrical approach so common today places extreme pressure on practitioners and fosters passivity in patients and families. Therapy or support groups for dying children and their families should be increased (Fllanagan 1933, Pakes 1983, Rolsky 1983); such groups could relieve or prevent suffering by providing information on health care procedures, opportunity for release of emotions, and a sense of group solidarity. Support groups for professionals could be an ongoing source of social solidarity and help prevent emotional problems like burnout (Pakes 1983, Wessels 1983).

PREVENTION OR AMELIORATION OF SUFFERING IN THE TRANSCENDENT DIMENSION

There are two principal themes in this dimension: "resilience" and "community." The bereaved can recover the lost parts of their personhood and become resilient at a more mature level of integration of self. Kliman (1968) noted that the majority of bereaved children have constructive-favorable outcomes following the death of a parent, which can lead to adequate functioning as well as growth toward personal identity. The experience of childhood bereavement can lead to the socially useful function of creativity and even to outstanding achievement in art, science, or politics. Binger, Ablin, Kushner, and Perin (1983) studied six families whose children with cancer had been cared for at home; they found that family members felt greater maturity and emotional growth because of the tragedy. Finally, constructing or developing a community of people who are concerned with childhood bereavement can provide a new, (secular) transcendent, meaningful sense of strength, belongingness, and positive self-evaluation within the context of social activism (Bensman and Rosenberg 1976, Cassel 1982, Kliman and Rosenfeld 1980).

REFERENCES

Albee, G. 1983. "Primary Prevention of Psychopathology." In R. Corsini, ed. *Encyclopedia of Psychology*, vol. 3. New York: John Wiley & Sons, pp. 67–69.

Albee, G. 1985. "The Answer Is Prevention." *Psychology Today* 19(2):60–64.

Bensman, J. and B. Rosenberg. 1976. *Mass, Class, and Bureaucracy: An Introduction to Sociology*. New York: Praeger Publishers.

Binger, C. M., A. R. Ablin, J. H. Kushner, and G. A. Perin. 1983. "Terminal Phase of Childhood Cancer: Home Care of the Dying." In J. E. Schowalter, P. R. Patterson, M. Tallmer, A. H. Kutscher, S. V. Gullo, and D. Peretz, eds. *The Child and Death*. New York: Columbia University Press, pp. 156–171.

Bowlby, J. 1980. Attachment and Loss, vol. 3 of *Loss*. New York: Basic Books.

Brofenbrenner, U. 1973. *Two Worlds of Childhood: U.S. and U.S.S.R.* New York: Touchstone Books.

Buckingham, R. W. 1983. "Hospice Care for the Dying Child." In J. E. Schowalter, P. R. Patterson, M. Tallmer, A. H. Kutscher, S. V. Gullo, and D. Peretz, eds. *The Child and Death*. New York: Columbia University Press, pp. 199–206.

Cassel, E. J. 1975. "Dying in a Technological Society." In P. Steinfels, and R. Veatch, eds. *Death Inside Out: The Hastings Center Report*. New York: Harper & Row, pp. 43–48.

Cassel, E. J. 1982. "The Nature of Suffering and the Goals of Medicine." *New England Journal of Medicine* 306:639–645.

Deasy-Spinetta, P. and J. J. Spinetta. 1983. "The Child with Cancer Returns to School: Preparing the Teacher." In J. E. Schowalter, P. R. Patterson, M. Tallmer, A. H. Kutscher, S. V. Gullo, and D. Peretz, eds. *The Child and Death*. New York: Columbia University Press, pp. 303–314.

Deutsch, H. 1975. "Absence of Grief." In A. C. Carr, B. Schoenberg, D. Peretz, A. H. Kutscher, and I. K. Goldberg, eds. *Grief: Selected Readings*. New York: Health Publishing Corp., pp. 191-201.

Feinberg, D. 1970. "Preventive Therapy with Siblings of a Dying Child." *Journal of the American Academy of Child Psychiatry* 9(4):644–669.

Flanagan, C. H. 1983. "Children with Cancer in Group Therapy." In J. E. Schowalter, P. R. Patterson, M. Tallmer, A. H. Kutscher, S. V. Gullo, and D. Peretz, eds. *The Child and Death*. New York: Columbia University Press, pp. 266–292.

Gelman, D., D. Shapiro, H. Morris, J. Shirley, E. Karagianis, and S. Katz. 1985. "Patient, Heal Thyself." *Newsweek* CV(12):82–84.

Grollman, E. a. 1967. "Prologue: Explaining Death to Children." In E. A. Grollman, ed. *Explaining Death to Children*. Boston: Beacon Press, pp. 1–27.

Jacobs, J. 1961. *The Death and Life of Great American Cities*. New York: Vintage Books.

Kliman, G. 1968. *Psychological Emergencies of Childhood*. New York: Grune & Stratton.

Kliman, G. 1969. "The Child Faces His Own Death." In A. H. Kutscher, ed. *Death and Bereavement*. Springfield IL: Charles C. Thomas, pp. 20–27.

Kliman, G. W. 1975. "Analyst in the Nursery: Experimental Application of Child Analytic Techniques in a Therapeutic Nursery — The Cornerstone Method." *Psychoanalytic Study of the Child* 30:472–510.

Kliman, G. W., and A. Rosenfeld. 1980. *Responsible Parenthood: The Child's Psyche Through the Six Year Pregnancy.* New York: Holt, Rinehart, & Winston.

Kübler-Ross, E. 1969. *On Death and Dying.* New York: Macmillan Co.

Liebow, E. 1967. *Tally's Corner: A Study of Negro Streetcorner Men.* Boston: Little, Brown & Co.

Lindemann, E. 1975. "Symptomatology and Management of Acute Grief." In A. C. Carr, B. Schoenberg, D. Peretz, A. H. Kutscher, and I. K. Goldberg, ed. *Grief: Selected Readings.* New York: Health Sciences Publishing Co., pp. 85–92.

Marten, G. W. and A. M. Mauer. 1983. "Psychosocial Interactions of the Dying Child, His Parents, and Health-Care Professionals." In J. E. Schowalter, P. R. Patterson, M. Tallmer, A. H. Kutscher, S. V. Gullo, and D. Peretz, eds. *The Child and Death.* New York: Columbia University Press, pp. 235–249.

Martinson, I. M. 1983. "Home Care for Children with Cancer." In J. E. Schowalter, P. R. Patterson, A. H. Kutscher, S. V. Gullo, and D. Peretz, eds. *The Child and Death.* New York: Columbia University Press, pp. 172–179.

Maslach, C. 1982. *Burnout — The Cost of Caring.* Englewood Cliffs NJ: Prentice-Hall.

McPheeters, H. L. 1977. "Mental Health Programs." *Proceedings of the Academy of Political Science* 32(3):1519–169.

Nieburg, H. A. and A. Fischer. 1982. *Pet Loss.* New York: Harper & Row.

Pakes, E. H. 1983. "Care for the Caregivers." In A. C. Carr, B. Schoenberg, D. Peretz, A. H. Kutscher, and I. K. Goldberg, eds. *Grief: Selected Readings.* New York: Health Sciences Publishing Corp., pp. 61–84.

Parkes, C. M. 1975. "First Year of Bereavement." In A. C. Carr, B. Schoenberg, D. Peretz, A. H. Kutscher, and I. K. Goldberg, eds. *Grief: Selected Readings.* New York: Health Sciences Publishing Corp., pp. 61–84.

Rolsky, J. T. 1983. "Helping a Child with Leukemia to Die at Home." In J. E. Schowalter, P. R. Patterson, M. Tallmer, A. H. Kutscher, and I. K. Goldberg, eds. *The Child and Death.* New York Columbia University Press, pp. 180–186.

Rosenfeld, A. 1976. "And Now, Preventive Psychiatry." *Saturday Review,* Feb. 21:24–25.

Silverman, A. 1984. "Pet Loss — A Teaching Model." *Archives of the Foundation of Thanatology: Euthanasia in Veterinary Medicine: Anticipatory Grief, the Euthanasia Process, Acute Grief and Bereavement — Including Implications for All Medical Disciplines,* #29. New York, Foundation of Thanatology.

Solnit, A. J. 1983. "Changing Perspectives: Preparing for Life or Death." In J. E. Schowalter, P. R. Patterson, M. Tallmer, A. H. Kutscher, S. V. Gullo, and D. Peretz, eds. *The Child and Death.* New York: Columbia University Press, pp. 1–18.

Steinmetz, Ross, E. 1967. "Children's Books Relating to Death: A Discussion" In E. A. Grollman, ed. *Explaining Death to Children.* Boston: Beacon Press, pp. 249–271.

Wessels, D. T., Jr. 1983. "Professional Burnout: An Issue for Those Treating Muscular Dystrophy Patients." In L. I. Charash, S. G. Wolf, A. H. Kutscher, R. E. Lovelace, and M. S. Hale, eds. *Psychosocial Aspects of Muscular Dystrophy: Commitment to Life, Health, and Function.* Springfield IL: Charles C. Thomas, pp. 84–91.

10

How Parents Can Help Children Cope with Death

Daniel Schaefer

Children are not attending funerals these days. By way of explanation, parents often say, "My kids are not exposed to death." But let us take a look at what is affecting children today. The TV, the radio, the newspapers are filled with stories of natural disasters, fires, airplane crashes, murders, suicides, assassinations. Death's presence is ubiquitous. But parents still say, "I've been able to protect my kids from death. They really don't realize what's going on."

Parents in crisis are the focus of my efforts as a funeral director. When I make funeral arrangements with them, they are often deeply distraught, struggling with the shock of a sudden death or exhausted by the ordeal of a relative's slow death. Communicating with their children makes them uncomfortable because they themselves are grieving. They are terribly stressed, they lack energy, and their attention span is reduced. Nevertheless, they are concerned about what effects the death will have on their children and want to protect them. These parents may be unprepared and lack information, but they are not unwilling to talk to their children.

Three years ago, I received a phone call in the middle of the night: my brother had been killed in an automobile accident, and I knew that at 7:00 A.M. I would have to tell my children that their uncle was dead. I said to my wife, "The unusual thing is that I know exactly what I'm going to say to the kids. I've written a book on the subject and I have all the information. But I still have a knot in the pit of my stomach. Can you imagine what it must feel like for someone who does not have the information and has to do the same thing?"

EXPLAINING DEATH TO CHILDREN

In the course of funeral arrangements, I help parents explain the death they are experiencing to their children. To do so does not require a long, drawn-out seminar or educational program. It only takes five minutes; the children's attention span is not longer. From each family's individual blueprint, I take the building materials available and I construct the message that will fit that blueprint.

Children who are sent away to someone else's house when a loved one dies become solitary mourners. They cannot handle all that is going on by themselves. I tell parents that they have a choice of making their children be "inside kids" or "outside kids." Inside kids are brought into the family support network and are given help, and outside kids are left alone. A friend tells the following story. He moved from the city to the suburbs at age nine. His grandfather died shortly after he moved, but he was not told of his grandfather's death until he was eleven yeas old — two years later. His parents made him an outside kid.

Parents must learn what kinds of questions to expect from their childen. They must not be surprised that children will connect events that may have no connection. If, for example, a parent says to a child, "Grandma had a pain in her stomach. She went to the hospital and she died," the child may think, "Gee, the next time Mother gets menstrual cramps, she is going to die." The child will become upset, and the parent will have no idea why. In another case, a parent will say, "Grandma died because she was very, very old." But children are concerned about the death of their own parents. One woman told me that her eleven-year-old daughter kept saying to her, "Please, Mommy, go get your hair dyed." Children sometimes think that old people die when their hair becomes gray. If their parents will dye their hair, they will postpone death for a while.

Children aged three to six years have magical, concrete thinking. How does a parent respond when a child asks, "How do dead people eat chocolate cake?" In fact, what the child is saying is, "Somewhere grandfather is still alive and if we could only get him the chocolate cake he likes, he would be able to eat it." There are many other examples of this kind of concrete thinking, but the fact is that young children think that death is reversible.

Not enough thought is given to how to handle teenagers when a death occurs. It would help if a parent said, "It's possible that you'll walk back into school and think you see your brother or hear his voice, or you won't be able to sleep." If a parent says these things to a child in advance, when such events happen the child is better prepared.

My program with parents in crisis is fourfold: coping with sadness, accepting death, understanding why the death happened, and explaining what will happen next. Why not say to a child, "Listen, the reason we're sad is because _____ died, not because of anything you did." Most kids will think that they are somehow responsible for whatever is going on. It is important that they understand what the sadness is about.

THE MEANING OF DEATH

What does it mean that someone is dead? One can give a basic biological explanation of death: when somebody dies, his or her body stops working and it is not going to work any more. This answers many questions. it is an explanation that parents can use as a foundation. They can come back to it on a regular basis. When a child asks, "How do dead people eat chocolate cake?" the parents can explain that dead people can't eat because their bodies aren't working any more — they can't eat chocolate cake or anything else. When a child says, "It's raining outside; is Grandpa's body going to get wet? Is he going to feel cold?" the parents can say, "No, he's not going to feel wet or cold because his body doesn't work any more. You can only feel if your body is working." This is something parents can use without wondering what they may have said the last time the child asked a question, or worrying that they may confuse the child.

Parents should give children an outline they can work with. They should tell them what is going to happen and bring them into the support network, not send them away from it. Encouraging parents to do so can take a lot of patience. I often have to point out the shortcomings of the explanations that parents have customarily used and remind them of the importance of honesty and clarity when talking to children.

THE FUNERAL

People can seldom get through a crisis without a support network, but the support network can also cause damage. For example, some people say, "Don't say anything to the child; don't bring the child to the funeral." They misunderstand grieving. For example, when one boy's father died a few years ago, the boy said, "I want to go play in the soccer game." I spoke with him about it. "If you want to go play in the soccer game, it's all right. Your father's wake is going to start at two o'clock. When you get to the game, some people may ask you how you could possibly be there, since your father just died." It is important for the child to know what to expect. Another example occurs when a child asks, "Why am I laughing when my father just died?" This question has to do with misunderstood grieving, as if bereavement were a period of unrelieved forced solemnity.

People often ask whether or not they should bring a child to the funeral. The answer is that they absolutely should not unless the child has been prepared beforehand and given enough information about what to expect. Then the child can be asked, "Do you want to come?" The child may say no or yes, but at least has been given the opportunity to choose.

People seem to need a license to grieve. Perhaps it should be like a driver's license, with a picture on it. A person could hold it up and say, "See, my grandfather died three years ago, and I have a license to feel dreadful today." Or, "My mother died a year and a half ago, and I'm still grieving. I have a license to do so, so please accept me this way." That is really what happens within the context of the funeral. People must be allowed to do what they want to do and what is important to them.

A fourteen-year-old boy who accompanied the adults of his family when they came to arrange his grandfather's funeral said, "I want to bury my baseball trophy in the casket with my grandfather." His uncle said in disbelief, "That trophy is four feet high and it's yours. Do you really want to part with it?" He answered, "Yes. It's my grandfather, and I want to bury the trophy with him." So it was done. This boy was strong and assertive enough to say, "I don't care what anyone says. If you will let me do it, then I am going to do it."

People sometimes come to me and say, "I want you to order flowers for the funeral, to be from my children." I reply, "Why don't you ask the kids what they want to do?" Children may come in with a handful of weeds from a garden, and those weeds are more significant to them than an expensive bouquet would be.

A mother may think, "I wish I had put the teddy bear in the casket with my baby, but nobody told me I could." Some mothers are not even aware that they can bury a stillborn or miscarried baby in a grave — a grave they can then visit and on which they can place flowers. When newborns die in a hospital, the hospital personnel often say, "Don't worry about it. The hospital will take care of the funeral: everything will be paid for." Later, the mother will ask, "Where do I go to put flowers on Mother's Day? Where is my baby buried? I don't even know."

CONCLUSION

A funeral is not like painting a room. A room can be painted blue one day and red the next day, but with a funeral, people have a limited period in which to decide what they want to do or what they feel is important. After that, they cannot do it over again. Therefore, it is a period when people have to consider carefully what they are doing. People may say, "Leave me alone. I don't want any of this psychological garbage. I'm too distraught at this point." Here it is appropriate for the funeral director to introduce the subject of the children. Nobody ever says, "I don't want to hear what you have to say to my children."

Then the funeral director must talk about anger, guilt, and responsibility. The adults generally do respond. Talking about teenagers allows discussion of how one can be angry at a funeral. It helps to talk about the guilt commonly felt by teenagers, how they may feel responsible, and so on. Talking about children to grieving parents helps them cope with their own grief.

11

Replacement Children

Sherry E. Johnson

This chapter describes my research and practice with fourteen couples, aged twenty-four to fifty-three, who had experienced the death of a child one or two years earlier and who then had subsequent children. For eight of the couples, the warning or preparation time before the child's death was fourteen days or fewer, and for six couples it was fifteen days or more. Of the children who died, there were seven boys and one girl in the short-preparation group and four boys and two girls in the long-preparation group. The causes of death included sudden infant death syndrome, heart disease or cardiac problems, anoxia, and leukemia.

The initial intent of the study was to explore the question of guilt feelings on the part of the parents. The issue of subsequent children arose in two areas of the research: (1) the suspension or the resumption of sexual activity after the death of the child and any guilt that was associated with it; and (2) how these parents made the decision to resume normal living, both as a couple and individually.

It should be pointed out here that the terms *replacement children* and *subsequent children* have different meanings. The conception of replacement children is a response to unresolved parental grief over the death of previous children. Such children tend to develop emotional problems. Subsequent children, although born after the death of a sibling, typically do not develop emotional problems because of the previous death. Not all subsequent children are replacement children.

REACTIONS TO THE CHILD'S DEATH

The child's death, as might be expected, was extremely traumatic for the parents, giving rise to a sense of emptiness (too much time on their hands and not enough activities) and feelings of loss of the love object, which were strongly associated with stress and feelings of guilt. Sexual intercourse symbolized the creation of the now-dead child and hence was terminated for some period after the death. Other factors that made sex unwelcome were (1) that it was not, in certain cases, an important part of the marriage; (2) that there were marital problems before the death; and (3) that several women were postpartum at the time of the child's death.

The couples believed that one way to fill the void in their lives and to alleviate their guilt was to create another child. Information about subsequent children continually evolved during the interviews, especially when the parents were asked if they had made a decision to go on living again. Once the parents had decided to have another child, sex became a welcome act, not chiefly for pleasure or comfort, but for procreation.

Most of the parents had another child as a means not only of beginning to live again but also of filling the void and alleviating guilt. They would say things like, "We have another chance: we'll be better parents this time." The need for another child and the guilt feelings associated with the child's creation have been reported in only a few other studies, which found that guilt may be transferred to and affect the subsequent child.

DEVELOPMENT OF EMOTIONAL PROBLEMS IN SUBSEQUENT CHILDREN

My research and practice suggests that once the child learns that there was a previous child, he or she develops what Lifton (1967) calls "survivor's guilt." Frequently, the subsequent child learns that the previous child had to die before he or she could be conceived or adopted. Therefore, the child may begin to express such ideas as "Why am I alive and my sister or brother dead?" "I feel guilty because I am alive and my sibling is dead."

An important issue in the development of emotional problems in subsequent children is related to how, when, and why the parents decided to have another child. My research revealed differences between the short-preparation group and the long-preparation group in this regard. Of the eight couples in the short-preparation group, four had a child within the first year of bereavement. Three couples were pregnant at the time of the interviews and one became pregnant soon after the interview. Two others had children early in the second year of bereavement. Six of the eight couples were therefore pregnant some time during their first year of bereavement.

One woman in the short-preparation group had physical problems and was advised not to become pregnant again; subsequently, she and her husband discussed adoption. This couple donated a grave and paid the burial expenses for an unidentified child who had been found dead in a garbage can. Soon afterward, they assumed the care of a foster child who had been diagnosed as having apnea (their own child had died of sudden infant death syndrome). This couple divorced during the second year of bereavement.

Another couple had a remaining newborn twin and chose not to have another child. Since that time, two other couples in the short-preparation group have each had a subsequent child.

The long-preparation couples were older than the short-preparation couples; three of them were no longer of childbearing age. One woman who was still of childbearing age had physical problems and believed that she should not become pregnant again; she therefore underwent a tubal ligation during the first·year of bereavement. Another couple had a baby in their first year of bereavement but in the second year were divorced. For the woman the trauma was compounded by her decision to have an abortion after her ex-husband had raped her. The sixth couple had had a child with spina bifida and were too frightened to have another baby who might be born with the same condition.

To summarize, two years after the death of the children, seven of the eleven childbearing couples had subsequent children and one had a remaining twin. Two couples did not have another child because of physical problems and one chose not to have another child for fear of the birth defect recurring. Also in the second year, two couples were pregnant with their second child since the death.

Although these couples understood that they could not replace their dead child, they wanted another child of the same sex and as quickly as possible. One couple had intercourse as soon as they returned from the hospital after learning that their child had died of sudden infant death syndrome. Couples, both in the study and my practice, have gone to great lengths to achieve the pregnancy. One father had a vasectomy reversed the month after his child had died; the subsequent child was born nine months later.

Several parents mentioned that they would like to give the next child the same name as the one who had died. None of them actually did so, but many parents, perhaps unconsciously, used a name with the same initial. If the subsequent child turned out to be the opposite sex of the child who had died, the parents were initially upset but decided they would "keep" the child.

Cain and Cain (1964) worked with disturbed replacement children at least eight to thirteen years after the death of the previous child. They discovered two important things about the parents of these disturbed children. First, the mothers were predominantly guilt-ridden, depressive, phobic, and compulsive, and had experienced many losses during their own childhoods. Second, these parents had an intense narcissistic investment in their dead children.

Lehrman (1956), Natterson and Knudson (1960), and Solnit and Green (1951) also reported pathology in parents who attempted to replace a child; the parents they studied were premorbid, phobic, obsessive, and depressive, or were older and found it difficult to raise a young child. In addition, these researchers found that excessive idealization of the dead child, the suddenness of the child's death, and the death of an older child increased the likelihood of emotional problems in replacement children.

Can parents of childbearing age who have lost a child have a normal need to bear and parent another child? If parents live for a child and that goal is extinguished, can they then replace that child without having a pathological outcome? And how can we, as clinicians, counsel parents who want and need another child so that the child will become a subsequent child rather than a pathological replacement child?

I am longitudinally following the subsequent children of the fourteen couples in this study to see what will happen in their lives. I have found some interesting variables that can affect the decision of parents to have another child. In assessing and counseling the parents, I have found that it is imperative to assess their resolution of grief and their mental health. The study by Cain and Cain (1964) reported that subsequent children were born into the world of mourning—of apathetic or withdrawn parents—a world focused on the past and on worship of the image of the dead child.

In my research, all of the parents who had a baby or who became pregnant in the first and second year of bereavement had made a decision to start living again. They did not exhibit apathetic or withdrawn behavior, although they still missed and grieved for their dead child. They had begun to fill the void that was left by the death and to reorganize their lives, certainly a primary task in bereavement. Although frightened of the unknown, all of them were nonetheless excited and pleased about their forthcoming children.

Another area to assess is the age of the parents. All of the parents in the Cain and Cain study (1964) were in their late thirties or early forties and were not prepared for a new baby in the home. That study implied that before the death of their child these parents had chosen not to have any more children. In addition, the children who died had been of latency age and early adolescence. In my study, all but one couple who had a subsequent child had been starting their families; their dead children had been between nine days and three years of age. Except for one couple, the parents were in their twenties and thirties. The older couple had two children, the youngest of whom was age three when he died. Previously, they had had no intention of having any more children, but the father had his vasectomy reversed after the child's death.

The third area that I assess is whose decision it is to have another child. Cain and Cain (1964) reported that it was the mothers' decision to have another baby and that the fathers were hardly involved in the decision. In my study, all but one couple had mutually decided to have a subsequent child; as for the couple who divorced in the second year of bereavement, the decision rested with the mother.

Ultimately, whatever the motives, it is the parents' decision whether to have another child; it is not and should not be the clinician's decision. Ethically, however, clinicians have an opportunity to help parents make an appropriate decision about having another child and to help them see the implications of this decision. It is hoped that they will come to realize that they cannot have another child to replace the one they lost but must, instead, learn to accept and love for its own sake the subsequent child whom they feel they want and need.

REFERENCES

Cain, A. and B. Cain. 1964. "On Replacing A Child." *Journal of American Academy of Child Psychiatry* 3:443–456.
Lehrman, S. R. 1955. "Reactions to Untimely Death." *Psychiatric Quarterly* 30:545–578.
R. J. Lifton 1967. *Death in Life: Survivors of Hiroshima.* New York: Vintage Books.

J. Natterson and A. Knudson. 1960. "Observations Concerning Fear of Death in Fatally
Ill Children and Their Mothers." *Psychosomatic Medicine* 22:456–465.

A. J. Solnit and M. Green. 1959 "Psychological Considerations in the Management of
Deaths on Pediatric Hospital Services. I. The Doctor and the Child's Family." *Pediatrics*
24:106–112.

12

Parents by Default: Grandmothers and Aunts Who Become Caretakers of Children Whose Mothers Have Died

Paul M. Brinich

The Childhood Loss Program (CLP) at University Hospitals of Cleveland was set up in 1983 to offer a variety of psychological services to children and families who had suffered losses because of separation, divorce, illness, and death. During its first 30 months, some 253 children were referred for services; of these, 145, or 57 percent, were referred following a death.

Among these 145 children were 47 whose mothers had died (from illness, accident, homicide, or suicide). Of these 47 children, 28 were placed with relatives after the death of their mothers. This report discusses some of the special clinical problems observed in this group.

BACKGROUND

The ages, sexes, and ethnic backgrounds of the 28 children appear in Table 1. The children ranged in age from three to 19 years, with no clear modal age. Fifty-four percent were male and 89 percent were black. The causes of death and the ethnic backgrounds of the 22 mothers are shown in Table 2. Illness claimed 41 percent, accidents 14 percent, homicide 41 percent, and suicide 5 percent. (There are fewer mothers than children because some of the children were siblings.)

The proportion of violent death (59 percent) among these mothers necessitates some comment. Although this figure may seem high, it is, unfortunately, not out of line with statistics collected by the U. S. Department of Justice (Langan and Innes 1985). It reflects the fact that the mothers were largely young, black, poor, and living in urban ghetto areas.

Table 3 shows the current living arrangements of the 28 children. Almost all (79 percent) were placed with female maternal relatives, who often took on the task of raising these children alone, without the support of a spouse.

Thus, we are dealing with children who have suffered multiple losses, including the death of their mothers, the loss (or absence) of their fathers, and subse-

TABLE 1

Age, sex, and ethnic background of maternally bereaved children
living with relative caretakers

Age	Sex			Ethnic Background		
(yrs)	Male	Female	Total	Black	White	Other
3		1	1	1		
6	2	1	3	2		1
7	2	1	3	2	1	
8	1		1	1		
9	1		1	1		
10	1	1	2	2		
11	1		1	1		
12		3	3	2	1	
13	1	1	2	2		
14	2	1	3	3		
15	1	1	2	2		
16	1	2	3	3		
17	1	1	2	2		
19	1		1	1		
Totals	15	13	28	25	2	1
Percent	(54)	(46)	(100)	(89)	(7)	(4)

TABLE 2

Cause of death by ethnic background for the mothers of bereaved children
living with relative caretakers

Cause of Death	Ethnic Background			Total	Percent
	Black	White	Other		
Illness	9			9	41
Accident	2	1		3	14
Murder 59%	8	1		9	41
Suicide	1			1	5
Totals	20	2		22	101
Percent	(91)	(9)		(100)	

quent out-of-home placement. These children usually come from chaotic families and are taken in by maternal relatives who have suffered losses in the death of the children's mothers. These relatives often receive little support for their efforts from the fathers of the children, from spouses, or from social agencies. It is not an encouraging situation.

TABLE 3
Placement of maternally bereaved children living with relative caretakers

Caretaker	Number	Percent
Maternal grandmother	10	36
Maternal great-aunt or great-great-aunt	2	7
Maternal aunt	9	32
Maternal cousin	1	4
Older sibling	3	11
Paternal aunt	3*	11
Totals	28	101

*This number represents three children from one family who were placed together with their paternal aunt.

AMBIVALENCE OF CARETAKERS

The title of this article refers to grandmothers and aunts as caretakers of these children. The word "caretaker" is misleading; the caretaking arrangements we describe are neither temporary nor limited to eight-hour shifts. Rather, these relatives are, in many ways, adoptive parents, although the formalities of adoption are rarely observed. (County welfare workers are only too glad when a family member offers to take in the bereaved children.)

Most of these caretakers were involved in the children's lives for years before the deaths that created their new roles. Thus, the children already had received a good bit of their "parental" care from these relatives. Even though these caretakers had experience with these children and the children often regarded them as quasi-parents even before the deaths of their mothers, the adjustment to the new relationship was rarely easy for either the caretakers or the children.

A frequent pattern is one in which the new caretaker is, on one hand, loving to the child and, on the other, rigid in the management of normal developmental issues. This behavior finds a complement, sooner or later, in the behavior of the child, who repudiates the care provided with statements like, "My *mother* wouldn't have done that!" or "I don't want to live here; I want to live with my auntie!" (or father or other relative).

A key to understanding the combination of love and rigidity in the caretakers is an appreciation of the anger that is also part of the relationship. This anger is related to the fact that these caretakers did not *choose* to become parents to these children; they were forced to step into the breach created by the death of the child's mother. Furthermore, the assumption of care for these children was usually costly for the caretakers. In every case we have seen, it has required major shifts in personal commitments and substantial financial sacrifices for the caretaker.

These adjustments had to be made against a background of personal mourning, for the dead mother of the child was also the daughter or sister of the caretaker. Matters seemed to be complicated further when the caretaker took responsibility for the child at the request of the dying mother. Some caretakers have said to the children "You know, I'd send you away in a minute, but I promised your mother I'd look after you." It is not hard to see the anger in such a statement.

Anger Toward the Dead Mother

The anger, which is directed toward the child, often has important connections to the dead mother. Whether or not the dead mother contributed to her own death (and in the majority of cases in this group she did), the caretaker felt angry toward the mother for having left her with the burden of the child. This anger was usually not acknowledged; if it appeared, it was in derivative forms such as "I know that she didn't *want* to die; she would have preferred to raise her child herself."

The mixture of loving and hating feelings toward both the child and the child's mother gets in the way of the caretaker's relationship with the child. The child usually requires a certain amount of flexibility in management, but the caretaker often feels stressed and angry and, therefore, is in a poor position to respond empathically and flexibly to the child's needs — needs that often have been amplified by the death of the child's mother.

Thus it was that a grandmother who was caring for a twelve-year-old boy whose mother had been stabbed to death forgot the circumstances of his mother's death when the boy was accused of pulling a knife on another child. Instead of seeing the anxiety that lay beneath the symptomatic action, she theatened to send him back to the neighborhood where his mother was killed (and where her killer is still at large). Thus it was that another grandmother who was caring for a three-year-old girl whose mother, during the year-long illness that preceded her death, had encouraged a great deal of regression in her daughter, was unable to see how this experience might play a part in the girl's separation anxieties. The grandmother tried to dismiss the girl's anxieties as silly worries. She did not see that when she told the girl "You can't keep hanging on me like this. I'm not going to be around forever!" she was not helping matters.

There is another source of anger toward the dead mother. Almost without exception, the caretakers of these children have expressed misgivings about the kind of care they received before the mothers died. Some of the mothers seem to have lived extremely disorganized lives, very much in contrast to the lives of most of the caretaking relatives. Other mothers, especially those who died after lengthy illnesses, seem to have regressed to childlike positions before their death and to have encouraged complementary regressions in their children. Thus, a caretaker may be faced with the problem of raising a six-year-old who thinks, feels, and acts as if he or she were three years old. The caretakers are, by and large, only too aware of these trends in the behavior of the mothers who died and left them to raise the children.

Identification

A final area of intense ambivalence in the caretakers has to do with the issue of identification. Many of the caretakers identified the children with their dead mothers. The question of whether or not the children are going to follow in their mothers' footsteps was not far beneath the surface in most of our cases.

Identification of the children with their fathers was also a problem, especially with regard to the fathers who had killed the mothers. The caretakers' concerns were shared by the children. Some children voiced worries that they would end up like their mothers. Others acted out, in a counterphobic way, the roles of victim and attacker. Still others developed somatic symptoms that mimicked those of their dead mothers.

Not all of the ambivalence was from the side of the caretakers, however. The children had their own inner conflicts with which to contend. For example, many of the children were consciously aware that with the deaths of their mothers their lives had actually taken a turn for the better. For the first time, there was some order in their lives. They were glad about this, but felt guilty for feeling so. It is easy to see how such guilt might link up with the feelings of guilty responsibility that are commonly associated with the death of a loved one. The guilt appeared to be especially intense when the children had felt a conflict in loyalties toward their mothers and their eventual caretakers while the mothers were still alive. Faced with such guilt, the children sometimes provoked rejection by their new caretakers.

Such responses are similar to what is known about the dynamics of adoptive families (see, for example, Brinich 1980, 1986). It is clear how a self-reinforcing cycle of loss, anger, internal guilt, external provocation, and mutual rejection can be started, especially given the warring feelings of love and anger that exist within the caretakers and the children. There are some points of difference, however, between these "families" and more usual adoptive families. First, these caretakers know a lot about the children's early lives; they also know that the children are, indeed, related to them by blood. These two factors limit (but do not elimiate) the tendency to "disown" conflictual aspects of the children — a tendency that is often seen in adoptive families. Second, all of these children knew their mothers and knew them well. The losses the children suffered in the deaths of their mothers were real. Those losses were also complicated by the fact that many of these mothers, for a long time before they died, had been unable, either physically or psychologically, to care for the children. This means that the children went into their new relationships with a great deal of unresolved ambivalence.

A third point of difference between these children and other adopted children is that most of these children knew their fathers and had mixed feelings about them. In several cases, it was the father who had killed the mother; in *all* the cases, the marital relationship of the parents had been troubled for years before the mother's death.

Finally, the relationships between these children and their caretakers often reflected the children's pervasive fear that their new caretakers also would die. Some children responded to this fear with inhibition; others seemed bent on constantly testing the limits of their caretakers' health and nerves.

CLINICAL ILLUSTRATION

A case drawn from our clinical practice illustrates many of the issues outlined earlier in this article.

The three A children—Barbie, Lonnie, and Robbie—were two, five, and seven years old when their mother became ill with congestive heart failure; she died about a year later. The children's father had been living with the family until his wife's illness. When she became ill, however, his problems with alcohol increased and the family broke up. Mrs. A took the childen to her mother's home and lived there until her death. When Mrs. A was on her deathbed, she asked her mother, Mrs. B, to take care of the chidlren. Mr. A went along with this request and voluntarily gave legal guardianship to Mrs. B after his wife died.

Mrs. B was in her mid-fifties when her daughter became ill. She was the oldest of several children and had raised her siblings when her own mother left home to escape an abusive relationship with Mrs. B's father. Mrs. B later married a man who, like her father, suffered from an addiction; she had many children by him before she finally divorced him. She raised her children alone, then began to work outside the home when she was in her mid-thirties; her last child left home when she was in her mid-forties. She was enjoying the greatest amount of personal and financial independence of her life when her daughter suddenly and unexpectedly became ill.

When Mrs. A died and left her children in their grandmother's care, Mrs. B was forced to quit her job and go on welfare so that she could care for the children. The youngest child, Barbie, was then three years old and responded to her mother's illness and death by becoming anxious about any separation from her grandmother. The middle child, Lonnie, age six, became enuretic, had frequent crying spells, and began to provoke fights in school. The eldest child Robbie was eight years old; he seemed withdrawn and passive, complained that he could not think in school, and worried about his own heart.

Mrs. B thought she was the best person available to take care of the children. She had been involved with their care before their mother's death, and her love for them was clear in the excellent care she provided for them afterward: they lived in a home where they were well fed, well groomed, and well dressed. This life was a contrast to the home life they had had while their parents were together; Mr. and Mrs. A had lived a chaotic life in which there were no regular meals, few restraints on the children's behavior, and constant anxiety about Mr. A's abuse of alcohol.

Mrs. B was aware of the changes that the children would experience when she took over their care. She was not happy that she now had to contend with the results of what she saw as her daughter's inability to stand up to her husband or to discipline her children. While she was sometimes able to recognize the strain that the losses and changes caused the children and how this strain was connected to some of their symptoms, she was more angry than she was understanding. Moreover, she was angry about the fact that, for the third time in her life, she was faced with raising several children with little or no support; she had become, at almost sixty years of age, a single parent with three young children.

Mrs. B sought the help of CLP about four months after her daughter's death. She was particularly concerned about how Barbie would "get up under her"; Barbie was always within an arm's length and insisted on sleeping with her arm around Mrs. B's neck. When the staff was able to be of some help with this first problem, Mrs. B mentioned her concerns about Lonnie and Robbie. The eventual treatment plan included Barbie's placement in a special therapeutic school, individual psychotherapy for both Lonnie and Robbie, and ongoing parental guidance for Mrs. B.

Parental guidance has been frustrating. Mrs. B often seems oblivious to some of her grandchildren's needs — those having to do with dependence, bodily contact, separation, and nurturance, all of which stem from the earliest years of childhood. Mrs. B is not really *oblivious* to these needs, she is *repelled* by them. The children make demands on her for a kind of responsiveness that she herself never received. It is as though a desperately thirsty woman has taken on the care of three children who are equally thirsty and who continually beg her to give them a drink. Their demands make Mrs. B more aware of her own thirst. When she pours out the few drops that she has, the children immediately demand more, and Mrs. B then explodes in anger.

One of the first things Mrs. B told me was that she was worried about how all three children seemed to want to cling to her. She made sure she sent them away on the weekends to one of her daughters; she wanted the children to realize that she "wouldn't be around forever." When Barbie began crying during one of her first visits to my office, Mrs. B threatened to put her in the bathroom down the hall and leave her there; she then turned to me and complained again about how Barbie clung to her every moment of the day.

Mrs. B was intensely angry with Mr. A. She thought that his inability to care for his wife during her illness had contributed significantly to her rapid decline and death. She was especially angry that when Mrs. A had lapsed into an irreversible coma and her doctor asked for permission to turn off the respirator, Mr. A was so drunk that he could not understand what was going on. Mrs. B had to intervene, putting pressure on Mr. A to consent to the turning off of the respirator. Finally, Mrs. B was angry that, since his wife's death, Mr. A had never offered any financial support for his children; he often did not even give them presents on birthdays or at Christmas.

Despite her anger at Mr. A and her knowledge that he was abusing drugs daily, Mrs. B allowed Mr. A to take the children to stay with him on weekends. She told me that she couldn't "take the children from him — they're all he's got." But Mr. A did not act as if he wanted the children. He did not come to pick them up when planned and then came unannounced on another day that suited his convenience. These visits to Mr. A's home did not stop until the night when Mr. A brought the children back at midnight, with the side of his car demolished, and was unable to tell Mrs. B how the car had been damaged.

Even now, Mrs. B is unable to tell Mr. A that if he wants to visit his children, he should tell them when he is coming and then live up to his promise, not just drop in whenever he feels like it. She is also unable to tell him to go away when he arrives drunk. (Mrs. B's difficulties in taking a firm stand with Mr. A have many links to her previous problems with both her father and her husband.)

As noted earlier, Mrs. B had special difficulty in managing some of Barbie's regressions, especially those related to separation. This difficulty seemed to be connected with Mrs. B's tendency to identify Barbie with Mrs. A. She says quite openly that Barbie looks just like her mother and sometimes she "forgets" that Barbie is not Mrs. A as a child. When Barbie and one of Mrs. B's adult daughters both claimed to have seen Mrs. A's ghost in the house, Mrs. B was caught between her wish that such contact might be possible and her generally firm belief that death is a boundary over which one cannot return. This makes it hard for her to help Barbie understand the "ghost" was not real, but the expression of a wish.

Mrs. B's tendency to identify Lonnie and Robbie with their father (Mr. A) has interfered with her ability to be a parent to them. When Robbie wanted to let his hair grow a bit (Mrs. B kept it cropped very short), she would not allow him to do so. It emerged that Mrs. B equated long hair with hanging around on street corners, with Mr. A, with drugs, and, ultimately, with an early death.

Mrs. B's ability to receive affection from these three children is sadly limited. When they make something for her, such as a Valentine's card, she accepts it but does not allow her pleasure to show. At the same time, she was furious when she saw Mr. A drop the card that Barbie had made for him onto the ground and leave it there as he stumbled out of the house. The only thing that makes her more angry is that all three children make a big fuss over their father whenever he drops in. She feels that she does the work while Mr. A collects the wages. She then feels that the children are completely self-centered and tells them that if they like their father so much, they should go live with *him*. Fortunately, the children are smart enough to reject this offer.

Our work with Mrs. B and the A children continues. Our hope is that we can help Mrs. B to recognize where some of her angry feelings belong and to limit the extent to which she displaces them onto the children. We also hope that we can help the children to avoid being pulled into a mutually provocative relationship with Mrs. B that would leave everyone feeling unhappy, angry, and rejected.

IMPLICATIONS FOR CLINICAL PRACTICE

Our clinical observations and data have several implications for clinical practice. Let us first look at the evaluation phase of this work and then move on to issues that arise in ongoing parental guidance. (Here I take for granted the principle that primacy of place goes to the development of a detailed understanding of the internal worlds of the bereaved children and those of their caretakers.)

Evaluation Phase

In this phase, we try to learn how the children and caretakers have woven the mothers' deaths (and all the preceding and surrounding events) into their internal models of themselves and of the world around them. Did they, realistically or not, play a part in the death? Have they understood it as a punishment? Do the children see themselves as destined to repeat their mothers' fate? Do the caretakers see the children as similarly doomed?

As far as the caretakers are concerned, we try to see what phase of their lives they were in when they took on this new responsibility. What adaptations have they had to make? What losses have they suffered beyond the death of a daughter or sister? What support have others given them as they have taken on these responsibilities? Did they wish to take on the task of childrearing or were they boxed into it by deathbed requests or by the limitations of other family members, such as the children's fathers, who would have been more appropriate to the task? Have the caretakers been able to tolerate and support the experience of mourning in themselves and in the children? Can they absorb some of the anger that bereaved children often experience without feeling personally attacked? Can they tolerate some of the children's feelings of attachment toward other family members without feeling rejected? And what are their own prior experiences of loss and bereavement? It is usually not possible to obtain the answers to all of these questions in a brief evaluation. This requires ongoing, long-term parental guidance.

In our experience, such parental guidance often returns to several themes. Prominent among them is the fact that the caretakers are parents by default; they did not want to take on the work, however much they might feel that it is their responsibility to do so. The grandmothers, especially, feel that they have already served their time, and the transition back to parenthood is difficult for them. Much of our effort is aimed at helping them find ways in which they can obtain some support and satisfaction while continuing to respond to the needs of the children.

Another prominent theme in parental guidance is the relationships between the caretakers and the dead mothers. As mentioned earlier, these mothers were daughters or sisters to the caretakers, and the caretakers naturally have intense feelings about them. It is important that the commonly encountered guilt about surviving the dead mothers and the anger at the mothers' dereliction of duty not be acted out toward the children. It is also important that the therapists not act out their anger toward the caretakers when the caretakers' own needs lead them to deny or neglect those of the children.

A third common theme is that of the relationships among the children, their fathers, and the caretakers. The caretakers often are angry at the children's fathers, whom they perceive as neglectful or, in some case, dangerous. It is hard for the caretakers to help the children come to terms with their ambivalent feelings toward their fathers, since the caretakers may become furious if the children show any signs of affection toward their fathers.

CONCLUSION

This chapter has described some of the problems encountered by grandmothers and aunts who take on the job of raising the children of their dead daughters and sisters. These problems center on the caretakers' ambivalent feelings toward the children, whom they love, and who love them dearly; toward the dead mothers, whom they love but who died and left them with the tasks of childrearing; and toward the fathers, whom they see as inadequate and neglectful or as murderous, depending on the circumstances of the mothers' deaths.

In our work with these caretakers, we attempt to help them recognize the sources of their ambivalent feelings and to limit the extent to which these feelings interefere with their ability to respond flexibly to the needs of the children. We hope that these preventive mental health services will keep the children and caretakers from falling into a cycle of loss, anger, guilt, provocation, and rejection that would make what is already a difficult adaptation into an impossible one.

REFERENCES

Brinich, P. M. 1980. "Some Potential Effects of Adoption upon Self and Object Representations." *Psychoanalytic Study of the Child* 35:107–133.

Brinich, P. M. 1986. "Adoption, Ambivalence, and Mourning." Paper presented at the annual meeting of the Northern California Regional Organization of Child and Adolescent Psychiatry, Carmel CA (January.)

Langan, P. A. and C. A. Innes. 1985. *The Risk of Violent Crime.* Washington DC: Bureau of Justice Statistics, U.S. Department of Justice.

13

Theoretical Perspectives on Suicidal Behavior in Adolescence

Marilyn M. Rawnsley

> There is but one truly serious problem and that is suicide. Judging whether life is or is not worth living amounts to answering the fundamental question of philosophy. All the rest...comes afterwards.
> — *Albert Camus*

Suicide strikes at the source of hope. Although the act of self-annihilation is at least as old as the dawning of human consciousness, the individual decision to self-inflict death still registers as dissonant, as a bizarre intrusion that disrupts some fundamental cosmic rhythm. Although the choice for death may be as impenetrable a human mystery as the instinct to survive against all odds, the latter occurs with such greater regularity that it is, if no less explicable, certainly less surprising. We can no more explain the will to live of one who has suffered a painful, disfiguring and isolating illness than we can the will to die of those who seemed no different from ourselves.

In the case of those who choose life, we posit an intuitive sense of hope; in the case of those who choose death, we hint vaguely at its absence. A simpler truth may be that our science lags behind our human experience. Our methods of inquiry, primarily designed to yield quantitative information on defined variables, may be inadequate to the task of understanding under what conditions people choose to live or die.

In this chapter, suicidal behavior in adolescents is viewed from a developmental premise and interpreted within five theoretical perspectives that suggest avenues for assessment and intervention. The theoretical systems were selected to provide a systematically derived eclectic framework for assessing adolescents at high risk for suicidal behavior. These five theoretical models are adapted from the sociological perspective of Durkheim (1951), the psychodynamic explanation as interpreted by Fenichel (1945), the learned helplessness model proposed by Seligman (1975), the crisis intervention approach described by Caplan (1964), the existential thinking of Binswanger (1958), and the interpretations offered by Neuringer (1962). The purpose of these models is to offer substantive explanations of the factors that may influ-ence adolescents' judgment of whether life is or is not worth living.

BACKGROUND

The less that is known about a phenomenon, the greater the speculation about its nature. The alarming increase in suicidal behavior among adolescents has provoked much speculation, but little explanation that can be useful in predicting, and thus preventing, the youthful decision to terminate an unfold-ing life. The inescapable and unacceptable fact that our children are killing themselves more effectively than any dread disease speaks eloquently, if tragically, to the urgency of developing strategies through which professionals and parents can recognize, reach, and appropriately refer young persons who are actively or potentially suicidal. This rising statistic has accentuated our concern about the lack of empirical knowledge of suicide, both completed and attempted. There is a recognized need for systematic investigation of the problem. The research findings to date are descriptive and inconclusive. Although such ambiguity may be appropriate when new understanding of a phenomenon is being sought, what clinicians need are theoretically derived models that can guide practice now.

Certain recurring themes have emerged in the data indicating those at high risk for potentially lethal behavior. Recent retrospective and cohort studies of adolescent suicide claim positive correlations between suicidal ideation, the expression of suicidal wishes, exposure to suicide, frequent use of alcohol and drugs, and previous nonlethal suicide attempts. As noted by one study group (Shafii et al 1985:1063), "clinicians and researchers have frequently debated whether or not those who commit suicide are different from those who attempt suicide or verbalize the wish to do so." The findings of these studies are of particular interest in dispelling such misconceptions. The data suggest that the behavioral patterns of adolescents at risk for suicidal actions are similar to those identified among adults: that those who talk about it and think about it are more likely to try it, that identification with or closeness to a suicidal victim increases suicidal potential, that use of alcohol and drugs diminishes inhibition of self-destructiveness, and that suicidal attempts of low lethality and other self-destructive behaviors merit assessment and appropriate interven-tion (Robbins and Alessi 1985; Shafii et al 1985). A plausible inference to be drawn from these data is that young persons who demonstrate any or all of the assessment characteristics could be considered as targets for professional intervention.

Given the complexity of the phenomenon and the scarcity of demonstrated preventive approaches, a multiple theoretical approach seems warranted. The substantive perspectives chosen illustrate diverse views of the problem of suicide. Durkheim's (1952) sociological typology of suicidal behavior as egoistic, altruistic, or anomic, postulated before the insights of psychodynamic theory, still has relevance for understanding an adolescent's self-destructive behavior within the context of the developmental task of establishing new social relationships (Durkheim 1952). Furthermore, the observation that Durkheim's position calls attention to suicide as a symptom of social tension and disease (Alvarez 1972), although beyond the scope of this discussion, may be pertinent to the rising incidence of suicide among American adolescents.

To a great extent, psychodynamic explanations of the meaning of suicidal behavior revolve around the psychoanalytic views expressed by Freud (1948) in his paper on "Mourning and Melancholia," in which he discussed the tendency toward suicide as sadistic behavior toward the self. However, Fenichel's (1945) discussion of suicide clarifies the psychodynamic changes that permit the punitive distortion of the superego/ego relationship. It is from Fenichel's discussion that the theoretical proposition and assessment characteristics in the psychodynamic model have been derived.

The third model is adapted from Seligman's (1975) work on learned helplessness. Although Seligman did not directly discuss active suicidal behavior, he clearly described the conceptual links between conditioned helplessness and depression. Since depression is postulated as a factor in suicidal and parasuicidal behavior (Emery 1983), a reasonable case can be made for a relationship between the factors associated with learned helplessness and passive or low-lethality suicidal attempts, which, either by design or accident, can result in death.

Crisis theory describes the conflicts of adolescence as a normal developmental process viewed within the context of the psychosocial environment. In discussing adolescent suicide as a response to developmental crisis, Gilead and Muhlaik (1983) focused on role change as the common stressor and cited research on diminished problem-solving and loss of significant relationships as precipitating factors. The crisis model presented here offers a broad interpretation of the construct of stressors from Caplan's (1964) original work. This model also incorporates the emphasis on problem-solving strategies and on establishing or maintaining adequate support systems as the goals of crisis intervention.

The final model is derived from an interpretation of the central theme of existential philosophy and psychiatry — that is, inauthenticity of self or failure to become the person one can be. Meaning in life occurs through participation in the existential struggle for authenticity or acceptance of responsibility for conducting one's life through decisions and choices. Neuringer's work (Bakan 1961) offers direction for understanding and answering the existential question "Why live?" that is compatible with a developmental perspective on adolescence.

Although the models are presented deductively — with the theoretical issues preceding the assessment of relevant factors and treatment approaches — in practice the selection of these theoretical sources proceeds inductively. Thus, the adolescent's behavior is assessed first and the conceptual focus is then contingent on the clinical judgment of its meaning. The models have therefore been constructed as a synopsis of the clinical process, from behavioral assessment to theoretical interpretation to treatment plan and evaluation (see Table 1).

Table 1. Five theoretical models of suicide.

Theory	Sociological	Psychodynamic	Learned helplessness	Crisis	Existential
Principle	Degree of individual integration in society	Intrapsychic energy, self aggression related to object loss	Degree of perceived self-competence in mastery of environment	Interaction between personal-environmental stressor(s) & resources	Phenomenological: the meaning and purpose of lived experience
Proposition	Discrepancy between role expectation and societal reward	Distortion of punitive superego on reality testing of ego	Outcomes are experienced as unrelated to behavior—i.e., uncontrollable	Disequilibrium between strength of stress and available resources	Awareness of responsibilities to act authentically in an indifferent world
Developmental premise	Adolescence requires contract with society that includes development of new social roles	Psychosexual state of adolescence demands mourning of original love object and re-investment of ego	Adolescence is a process of testing out new relationships between self & world that requires confidence in own abilities	Adolescence is an intensified maturational transition that introduces new challenges to coping	Adolescence begins the quest for universal significance of individual existence
Assessment characteristics	Egoistic: non-identified with values of peers or primary group; altruistic: completely absorbed in the values and identity of the group;	Death as fantasy of gratification; anger turned inward to punish others through self; depression as unresolved or delayed mourning for symbolic loss;	Motivation deficit: reduced initiation of responses; impaired cognition; interfering expectation that response cannot influence outcome; heightened emotionality;	Distorted perception of events; ineffective coping strategies; inadequate support systems; and increased developmental and situational stressors	New freedom & blurred values; existential anxiety, aloneness, purposelessness; fatalism—all-or-nothing dichotomy; high ideals and expectations of self

	anomic; rapid shift in social position; no referent group	desire and fear of independence	conditioned helplessness		
Goals and interventions	Promote adaptive social integration with peer and primary groups through peer group counseling, school activities, family therapy	Redirect aggression and build self-esteem; individual psychotherapy for corrective emotional experience to allow mourning and motion towards independence	Reduce cognitive & motivational deficits; behavior modification to set response/outcome contingencies including reality testing & feedback	Strengthen internal & external resources; short-term therapy to teach problem-oriented coping and identify environmental supports	Encourage decision towards responsible stewardship for own life; confrontation in supportive humanistic encounter with therapist and peers
Evaluation of outcome *Successful:*	Participation in appropriate and constructie age-related social activities	Redirection of aggression; sense of control	Increased perception of control & willingness to engage in new behaviors	Evidence of growth through improved coping strategies	Choice to continue living
Inadequate:	Increased social isolation from adults and peers	Parasuicidal and suicidal behavior, chronic depression	Increased sense of vulnerability, withdrawal and depression	Regression or consolidation of pattern of non-effective coping	Further detachment, despair and death

In no way are these explanations intended to be inclusive or conclusive. There are many theoretical perspectives on human behavior that could serve as a basis for the derivations of logically consistent propositions about suicidal behavior in adolescents, the suggestion of appropriate goals and treatment, and the initiation of research questions. The models in this chapter have been presented simply as examples of ways to proceed in interpreting and applying theory to practice when the need to provide reasoned responses to a problem far exceeds the empirical knowledge available.

SUMMARY

The incidence of suicidal behavior in adolescents should force us to re-evaluate our memories and myths about that turbulent transitional phase. Adolescence is the best and worst of times; it is soaring energy chained by social impotence; it is the struggle for personal identity curbed by conformity to the code of the group; it is the urge of intimacy confounded by the fear of rejection.

But we tend to rewrite the past. When we recall our own adolescence, we focus on its delights, the sexual stirrings framed in innocence, the opening up of the world without and within, the changes, the choices, and the freedoms. We project our fantasies on those who are adolescents now. The uneasiness that arrived with the awareness that we were mortal, that our promise was limited, that our love not always returned, that grownups were disappointingly flawed and could not always shield us from or guide us through life's losses, and that some dreams remain forever out of reach—all this we do not tell them, for we do not tell ourselves. Through the intervening years of adulthood, we have selectively maintained the souvenirs of our youth, saving the pleasures and discarding the pains. And despite our children's self-destructive behavior, which testifies to the high cost of our illusions, we seem to prefer our version of the truth.

To the extent that the pervasiveness of the problem is acknowledged, the theoretical perspectives presented here will be of use in identifying and helping young people who are at risk for life-threatening behavior. Systematic research that addresses both qualitative and quantitative aspects of self-destructive behavior will be sponsored to the extent that the public is willing to disarm its psychological defenses. We must recognize that our children are dramatically asking us for our protection and our help.

For those who have worked with or known adolescents or others who have chosen the ultimate violent separation of suicide, the need to promote prevention is particularly acute. The legacy of the suicide is confusion and pain. Estranged in death as they were in life, suicide victims haunt the shadows of memory. Restless and unforgiving, within us they do not rest in peace.

REFERENCES

Alvarez, A. 1971. *The Savage God, A Study of Suicide.* New York: Random House.

Bakan, D. 1961. "Suicide and the Method of Introspection." *Journal of Existential Psychiatry* 2(7,Fall): 313–322.

Binswanger, L. 1958. "The Case of Ellen West." In R. May et al., eds. *Existence.* New York: Simon and Schuster, pp. 237–364.

Camus, A. 1958. *The Myth of Sisyphus.* New York: Vintage Books.

Caplan, G. 1964. *Principles of Preventive Psychiatry.* New York: Basic Books.

Durkheim, E. 1951. *Suicide.* New York: Macmillan.

Emery, P. 1983. "Adolescent Depression and Suicide." *Adolescence* 27:70 (Summer), 245–257.

Fenichel, O. 1945. *The Psychoanalytic Theory of Neurosis.* New York: W. W. Norton and Co.

Freud, S. 1948. "Mourning and Melancholia." *Collected Papers,* vol. 4. London: Hogarth Press, pp. 152–170.

Gilead, M. and J. Muhlaik. 1983. "Adolescent Suicide: A Response to Developmental Crisis." *Perspectives in Psychiatric Care* 21:70 (Summer), 245–257.

Neuringer, C. 1962. "The Problem of Suicide." *Journal of Existential Psychiatry* 3:9, (Summer-Fall), 69–74.

Robbins, D. and N. Alessi. 1985. "Depressive Symptoms and Suicidal Behavior in Adolescents" *American Journal of Psychiatry* 142:5(May), 588–592.

Seligman, M. 1975. *Helplessness. On Depression, Development, and Death.* San Francisco: W. H. Freeman.

Shaftii, M., S. Carrigan, J. R. Whittinghill, and A. Derrick. 1985. "Psychological Autopsy of Completed Suicide in Children and Adolescents." *American Journal of Psychiatry* 142:9 (Sept), 1061-1064.

14

Adolescent Depression and Suicide

Samuel C. Klagsbrun

Thanks to recent studies, we know a great deal more today about the profile of the adolescent who commits suicide than we have known before. David Shaffer and colleagues have recently compiled such a profile. More males commit suicide than females. Young white men commit suicide in significantly greater numbers than do their black counterparts. Firearms commonly are used by substance abusers. Hanging is more prevalent in males, and jumping from high places for females. In attempted suicides, drugs are the most prevalent means.

A number of other conclusions culled from the body of recent suicide literature by Shaffer and colleagues include the statement that instances of the "copycat" phenomena do exist, as well as evidence that formerly hospitalized patients, both adults and adolescents, have a much higher rate of suicide than people who have never been patients. The data further suggest that symptoms of severe depression are the best predictors of later suicide. Suicide in adolescents takes place most often in the context of an acute disciplinary crisis or after an episode of rejection and humiliation immediately preceding the suicide.

Fifty percent of the patients who attempt suicide have had previous contact with mental health professionals. Diagnostic categories applied to the suicide include depression, antisocial behavior, drug and alcohol abuse, learning disorders, as well as anxiety, perfectionism, and (with a small number) manic-depressive illness or psychoses. Many of the people who have committed suicide have significant relatives with a history of attempted or actual suicide.

Finally, on the treatment side, the review of the literature indicates that those people who made repeated suicide attempts were found in greater numbers among patients given no follow-up appointments compared to those who used follow-up appointments given. The better results among those who had made suicide attempts took place in the population who had experienced short inpatient stays; in addition, the better results following suicide attempts were present among patients who were involved with programs having a very strong outreach component.

This, then, is a brief summary of the current state of knowledge based on 1) a survey of the literature on suicide, and 2) a major suicide research project of the Columbia University Department of Psychiatry.

But in this review of the subject, as is true of every investigation, it is the question we ask which determines the answer. Should the question be to identify the characteristics of suicide, the immediate precursors, the demographic profile, and the social context within which a suicide takes place? Or should it be to identify those factors affecting the sense of self present in the suicidal or depressed adolescent? If a question is raised addressing the factors which differentiate the depressed adolescent from his non-depressed counterpart, and if that question embraces those aspects of their history, their early experiences, and the society they live in, we may find fruitful areas of investigation begging for attention.

So far the characteristics identifying the depressed and suicidal adolescent have more to do with external circumstances and less to do with the person's inner life. I always tend to emphasize those factors relating to the environment, the upbringing, and the psychological set of mind of an adolescent who is depressed as more significant than the immediate circumstances preceding an actual suicide or suicide attempts. In exploring this subject, I deliberately exclude genetic, constitutional, or neurophysiological influences upon adolescent depression, since I believe that biological factors account for only a small percentage of adolescent depression and suicide. I also feel that in our present state of knowledge the treatment of such depression is misguidedly thought to be helped, if not cured, by a biological or medication approach as an answer to the problems of adolescent life. I choose in this presentation to set that part of the treatment spectrum aside and leave it to those people who enjoy basic sciences.

I may as well identify one other bias that I am certainly guilty of. I believe that treatment relating to life events which influence and have an impact on us must deal with our relationship to those events. Who we are as people, whether young or adult, and what we bring to those life events requires a treatment approach encompassing the person and those events. Frankly, not only do I not apologize for that viewpoint, but I think it is high time that those of us who take a sophisticated and sensitive philosophical stance towards living ought to become more articulate and aggressive in fighting against the reduction of life experiences to neurophysiological phenomena. We are human beings, we have a soul, we have aspirations, and we are truly more than a compilation of chemical reactions. I derive this view of us not from Carl Gustav Jung, who is a bit too mystical for my taste, but from a much more down-to-earth philosopher, my grandmother. She had a healthy disrespect for doctors, and even less respect for medications. On those occasions when she would experience a headache, she would take one aspirin, cut it in half, and then bite a tiny end of that half off, feeling very suspicious of what she had just ingested. She died smiling at the age of 87. After this overwhelmingly scientific introduction, let us turn to the matter we face.

The questions we have raised are chiefly environmental, questions of life experiences which adolescents face. Is there anything different in this generation's experience of adolescent life compared to that of previous generations? Is the increase to 5,000 deaths a year we have identified a transient phenomenon, or is it simply more accurate reporting? Is it a warning signal to all of us? Because if indeed our adolescents are killing themselves more frequently than ever before, and if by extrapolation the number of adolescents who are depressed is also much higher than ever before, then what kind of adults will soon be populating our world? Will their relationships be different? Will their commitment to the future be different? Will their sense of idealism and willingness to work to achieve those ideals be different? In short, will the culture of our society shift in a direction which may be deeply worrisome? Should we expect to face a significant increase of nihilism? Why this increase in adolescent death and depression, and what in our culture today might explain it?

Adolescents we have worked with for the last 11 years at Four Winds Hospital in Katonah, New York have left a definite impression on us. Let me present some thoughts based on those impressions. Our depressed and suicidal adolescents seem to me to present themselves as rootless, uninvolved, uncommitted, aimless corks bobbing up and down on the waves; and those characteristics seem to have been present in their lives for quite some time. As a group they are remote from their families, and they are cold. They band together in groups not out of friendship or even companionship, but more as predators seeking some constant outlet for a need to experience the passage of time in a way which would offset the boredom they feel. The group becomes a functional way to bring that about. An individual's involvement in any particular group is shallow and ephemeral. Young people in these groups are virtually interchangeable.

In this population, time does not exist. There is no past; there is no future; there is only the moment. There is flatness, an absence of feelings and emotions. The basic outward expression of emotions is the shrug. There are few facial expressions. Ironically, there is even an absence of sadness. What there is a lot of is emptiness.

The image I'm evoking is that of an adolescent removed from connections to emotions, except those having to do with momentary excitement. Surrounding such an adolescent with people and emotions, expecting to make a connection, is therefore not likely to have any impact. This adolescent does not necessarily have any particularly traumatic history. (Indeed, to the extent that one can ascribe this sense of vacancy to a specific event or series of experiences, the job of treating such an adolescent becomes significantly easier.) The image I have described seems akin to that of a concentration-camp survivor made numb and almost non-human by relentless exposure to traumatic events. There is a clue in that image and that association. Those of us who have worked with concentration-camp survivors have had the unnerving experience of knowing that silence is the survivors' most common response to inquiries about their history. It took approximately a generation and a half, 30 years after the end of World War II, for some of the early studies of the impact of concentration-camp experiences to begin to find their way into the psychiatric literature in some consistent way. It's as if the passage of a great deal of time was required before words could break the silence surrounding those experiences. A great deal of distance from those events was necessary before they could again be approached. The deep freeze which was the concentration camp experience trapped everyone who was caught in a condition beyond words. This is true even for adults who, on entry, had at least developed a vocabulary of life to take with them into the freezer. Even those people afterwards could not speak. The young people, the children who survived in those camps, had precious little vocabulary to start with when those atrocities overtook their young lives. When they came out, they came out scarred and mostly unable to articulate much of their experiences. Thirty years later, when the thaw finally occurred and the words began flowing, they came from people who felt that they had a responsibility to express something of that era and of their experiences in it. The people with a purpose spoke. Those who continued to feel empty continued to remain silent.

Adolescents who are depressed seem for some reason to be caught in a similar deep freeze. They are emotionally stunted, they are wordless, and they see their experience as pointless. They have been overwhelmed for too long by factors beyond their control. They seem to have very little to draw on in their short histories, and they certainly don't see a point to describing what it's like to people from whom they feel so alienated.

If this portrait of adolescence has meaning, it is because there are clues in the similarities and associations which offer us some insight. Perhaps we can take a bit of what we have learned from concentration camp survivors and apply those lessons to our adolescent survivors. But isn't that an extreme comparison to make, you may ask? Our adolescent survivors? Survivors of what? What is so terrible about the life of our adolescents to make them so turned off? In the age of endless TV, with multiple channels, what could be so awful about their experiences? Or as one kid said to me about his visit to London with his family, "How can a kid grow up there? It's abnormal! They only have four channels, and by midnight they're all closed down."

The impression I have of the quality of life available today to many adolescents is characterized by the shallowness of personal involvement of consistent adult figures in their lives. In the days of extended families and of significantly less mobility of people in those families, the number of solid, ever-present adults involved in the lives of adolescents, whether these adults were aunts, uncles, cousins, grandparents or neighbors, was a constant feature of everyday life.

Security for all of us is made up of a series of images and experiences deeply imprinted in our minds, which can always be counted on as a model of stability and constancy. Our extended families of old had enough presence day in and day out in our lives to stand for home. There was no nuclear and there was no extended; there was simply the family. The teachers who were part of our elementary school life for what seemed to be an eternity (because they had always been in that same school system), would always be there because they were never going to die. They, too, added to our sense of security, spanning years and reaching always into the future. That kind of stability, by the way, had very little to do with rich or poor, black or white. It was the basic stability of the neighborhood nourishing our sense of belonging, making us feel rooted.

Stability also means an ability to develop, hold on to, and depend on relationships which, predictably, will always be there. In order to develop basic primary attachments, one needs the stability of people and the circumstances around those people towards whom those attachments can develop. And so the basic ingredient which I feel is missing in society today, more than ever before, is the kind of life which allows for attachments to develop. When the absence of those qualities strikes a youngster at an age when he is unable to develop ways to compensate for that absence of stability, the damage created can be lifelong and severe.

What I hear from our patient population leads me to think about basic insecurity, about an absence of a certain kind of nurturing, about instability; and consequently about the tremendous importance of constant faces and places present over a long time. This constancy is primary requirement for a young person's ability to develop an identity which then has the capacity to develop relationships, to endure hardships, to have a sense of future, and a commitment to it. When those ingredients in life are absent or present only to an insufficient degree, we see the damage caused.

A depressed adolescent, as described before, is a numb person, unrelated, unconnected, having no sense of future or past. A depressed adolescent is ahistorical. Our experience in tracing the history of such adolescents repeatedly brings us to an awareness of a lack of connection to parents, an instability and lack of foundation in life, a feeling of not mattering to anyone precisely at a time in life when they are experimenting with a reaching out towards independence, which paradoxically requires even more of a secure foundation in family life and structured routines than ever before. When there is no one there, or when the family that is there is destructive, the foundation of the adolescent will not take shape and become a support. It is then that the factors described at the beginning of this chapter, the characteristics present in adolescent suicide, take over. A humiliation, a defeat, a crisis, a disappointment, all of these will precipitate a behavior which had its roots in the absence of a secure foundation for quite some time prior to the event.

To the extent that the treatment of a concentration-camp survivor ought to be based on a nonverbal approach, (because words are not available to that survivor), that treatment ought to include the structuring of activities, developing of routine behavior patterns, establishing once again to the extent possible regular relationships with the same faces, the same environment, the same plan for each day as a means of rebuilding foundations. So must it be for the depressed adolescent, because without that pattern, there is no way to plant one's feet in the present in order to reach for a future. To the extent that one can create regularity, which then allows for predictability, can one move slowly into the use of words. Security is preverbal. Once security is present, words may follow.

Our experience in treating the depressed patient, and certainly the suicidal patient, teaches us to recognize that an approach which initially de-emphasizes words and emphasizes stability in a structured environment has a good chance of succeeding. All this must be done over sufficient time to bring about the beginning of the thaw, indicated by the expression of subtle signals of trust and a wish to be involved in a relationship with the available, same, ever-present faces and people. Time is a crucial factor in the treatment for this group of patients. Do not be fooled by the short-term results of short-term therapy. Nurturing is the essence of what needs to happen during that time. The sense of continuity — of faces, environment, and concrete objects — is an essential requirement for success. In time, if enough nurturing and sameness is present, the greater the likelihood of a channeling of feelings and experiences into words.

Why are words so important? The Book of Genesis answers that in a unique way. According to the Bible, the first command God gave to Adam after God had created the world and all the things in it was to call upon Adam to give a name to every creature he saw. Without the spoken word, without the name, without a vocabulary and a language, there is chaos and disorder. Using words allows us to organize ourselves not only in relation to the world around us, but also in relation to our own internal world. Images alone are not sufficient. Language gives us the opportunity to plan and move ourselves through time. It is true that an enormous amount of preparation is required to bring to this point a depressed young person who had given up involvement in the world around him. But once that person chooses to use words, therapy can truly begin.

15

ASAP: Adolescent Suicide Awareness Program

Diane M. Ryerson

The Adolescent Suicide Awareness Program (ASAP) began in 1980. At that time, there were no effective suicide awareness and prevention programs such as ASAP would become. The alarming number of adolescent suicides called for the development of solutions, and "suicide prevention" became a major public health priority as experts searched for the knowledge and skills to stem this "disease."

In the absence of experts on adolescent suicide prevention, the staff at South Bergen Mental Health Center started to develop a program that would be educational and preventive — rather than reactive — to immediate tragedies. There were many hurdles to overcome in starting such a program. For example, there is often a pervasive, community-wide "cover-up" of many suicides, particularly those of young people. This cover-up is not done with any evil intent. Many times, law enforcement, medical, and judicial authorities declare a sudden and violent death to be an "accident" — when in fact probably was a suicide — in order to "spare" family and friends the agonizing legacy of a suicide.

As a rule, communities and schools do not openly address the problem of adolescent suicide until *after* one or more tragic deaths have occurred. Once a school or community is forced to confront the self-inflicted death of a student, there is a desperate scramble to assist teachers to cope, to reassure parents, and to inoculate students against future attempts.

A community typically uses several crisis-intervention approaches after it honestly and accurately recognizes that the death of one of its teenagers was a suicide:

1. An "expert" is invited to address an assemblage of parents, teachers, and, occasionally, students, in a large, impersonal meeting.
2. A brief discussion of suicidal behavior is held in a classroom of frightened students by a teacher who is unqualified to speak on the subject and who often has been ordered to perform this distasteful task.

3. A local mental-health worker is invited to address individual classes on the subject of suicide at the discretion of a teacher.
4. An informal support group is formed for the close friends of the deceased student.

These efforts are always well intended and may provide some help, albeit minimal, to those affected by the suicide. They may also reduce the risk of additional suicides in the community. They suffer, however, from three serious weaknesses. First, they always deal with a crisis. After a suicide, guilt feelings and sorrow are intense, and there is a high degree of resistance to suicide awareness programs, which often are seen as "too little and too late." Second, such efforts address the symptoms rather than the causes and usually do not expose the underlying problems. Third, and perhaps most important, these programs reach only a small portion of the community. Many parts of the community are left unaware of the critical warning signs and prevention strategies. These brief, one-shot affairs do not leave ongoing programs in place or create links among the school, community, and mental-health resources.

RATIONALE AND OBJECTIVES OF ASAP

My colleagues and I believe that each person in a school community needs to become knowledgeable about depression and self-destructive behavior in teenagers:

Educators need to know because they are in a unique position to identify and refer students who are at risk. Individual classroom teachers have extensive experience with "average" adolescents and have studied adolescent development during their training. They have daily contact with the same students, which enables them to compare the students' behavior. Furthermore, they are less defensive than parents and are not constrained by the strictures of peer loyalty to keep a suicide or a suicide threat confidential.

Parents desperately need this information because their children's lives are at stake. Parents are often inexperienced with or ignorant about the emotional difficulties of adolescents. Reluctant to acknowledge emotional difficulties in their own children, they frequently deny the seriousness of a teenager's despair until too late. Parents also need to know how to counsel and support their children when the children's friends are depressed and potentially suicidal.

Students need to have information about suicide, which could be a matter of life and death for them or for a friend. Teenagers have little experience with life and few well-developed coping skills. They do not realize that the feelings of depression they experience are usually time-limited and not a sign of inadequacy or mental illness. Since another student is the most frequent confidant of a suicidal peer, teenagers should learn to recognize the warning signs and know when, how, and where to get professional help. They need to learn that it is essential, sometimes even life-saving, to break a suicidal confidence.

On the basis of this rationale, we determined that our first goal would be to develop and maintain close, effective communication and referral procedures between the educational and mental-health systems.

The secondary goals of ASAP evolved when the pilot program was developed and field tested. They focused on major attitudinal changes that we believed were necessary if the program was to be effective in achieving the primary goals. They were

1. to detoxify attitudes toward emotional illness;
2. to demonstrate that psychotherapists are caring, knowledgeable, and approachable professionals to whom one can turn for help with an emotional problem; and
3. to reduce the reluctance to seek help.

KEY INFORMATION

We identified six key points that everyone in a school community needs to have for the school to become a prevention-oriented system: the warning signs, the facts about adolescent suicide, depression in adolescents versus staff, the causes of adolescent suicide, ways one can help, and sources of referral.

The Warning Signs

Most suicidal adolescents are ambivalent about their wish to die, wavering between longing to live and hoping to die. This ambivalence manifests itself in a range of verbal, behavioral, and symbolic warning signals that may be identified before a suicide attempt is made. Many caring, sensitive people, however, either overlook key signals or are reluctant to recognize such behavior as self-destructive, for fear of embarrassing the teenager or angering his or her parents. All participants need to examine the troublesome questions of when distressing behavior in a teenager is just "a phase" and when it indicates a risk of suicide.

The Facts About Adolescent Suicide

A thorough and accurate knowledge of the facts about adolescent suicide helps all members of a school community to appreciate the seriousness of the problem and to reduce the typical reaction that "suicide doesn't happen here." A frank discussion of these facts eliminates many misconceptions about suicide and reduces the taboo about confronting the problems openly.

The most common and troublesome myth about discussing suicide with teenagers, expressed by educators and parents alike, is the fear that if you talk about suicide with adolescents you may "put the idea in their heads" and motivate them to make a suicide attempt. Yet, the most common myth voiced by teenagers is the belief that suicide is somehow a romantic or heroic act and that to break the confidence of a suicidal friend is an unforgivable betrayal.

Young people need to know clearly that death is final and that when you are dead you cannot benefit from other people's sorrowful or remorseful reactions to your demise. Therefore, each group of participants in ASAP receives specific information about

- the annual number of adolescent suicides nationwide, statewide, and locally,
- the recent rate of increase or decrease,
- which groups of adolescents are at high risk for suicidal behavior,
- how many suicide attempts are made in relation to completed suicides, and
- the relation of suicide to other causes of adolescent deaths.

Depression in Adolescents

Many concerned adults misjudge the severity of an adolescent's depression and suicidal potential because they tend to evaluate the teenager by the same criteria they would apply to an adult suffering from depression. This is often a fatal mistake. To avoid tragic misunderstanding, parents and educators need to

- learn to review the developmental tasks and stages of adolescence;
- understand that distressing but not unusual life events — the breakup of a brief romance, academic failure, acute social embarrassment, or the loss of a family member by death or divorce — may precipitate a suicide attempt; and
- understand that adolescents are most concerned with the present, have difficulty comprehending that things will get better, and are often impulsive in their attempts to cope with pain.

Students also need to be alert to what might go wrong in a friend's (or their own) life that might create vulnerability to depression and lead to self-destructive impulses. Adults and teenagers alike should know that suicide does not strike randomly or suddenly but is the final common pathway for a series of life events, recent losses, and personality vulnerabilities. Suicide is an act, not a disease.

The "Causes" of Adolescent Suicide

Because the facts about many teenage suicides are shrouded in secrecy and denial, many people believe that self-destructive behavior strikes out of the blue. The complicated web of causative factors, as well as the warning signs, is unknown by key people who deal daily with teenagers. Entire school communities need a basic understanding of how certain past experiences and environmental conditions, personality vulnerabilities, and recent precipitating events can combine to place a despondent teenager at high risk of suicidal behavior.

How One Can Help

Again, all members of a school community need to know what to do and what not to do if they suspect that a young person may be considering suicide. People who are unsure of how to intervene may deny or overlook even blatant clues. Students, teachers, and parents need a series of simple, discreet steps to follow if they have reason to suspect suicidal intent. Specific strategies for the referral and management of a depressed teenager must be designed and used by each individual school system. Everyone needs to know the following:

- to whom in the school a potentially suicidal student should be referred;
- how the referral should be made;
- alternative procedures to use if the designated school official is unavailable or the need arises during a holiday;
- how the information will be used and by whom; and
- what further involvement — if any — the referring person should have with the troubled student.

These specific guidelines will reduce the anxiety and distress that most people experience when approaching a depressed teenager. Educators need reassurance that their administrators will support their intervention with troubled students. It is not unusual for a teacher to be concerned about the possible negative reaction of the school and parents to their "misidentifying" a potentially suicidal student. A specific set of procedures will reduce the reluctance of teachers to reach out to teenagers who need their help.

Sources of Referral

Each school system needs to identify the referral sources that are available in the community. Everyone should know

- how to contact a mental health agency twenty-four hours a day;
- what will happen when the contact is made;
- how to get professional help for a suicidal person; and
- how the referring person can render additional assistance and what type of help he or she can give.

Each school — public, private, and parochial — has specific internal referral sources. These sources range from a full child study team of professional social workers and psychologists, substance abuse counselors, and guidance counselors in a large public school to a single grade-level advisor or dean of students in a small private or parochial school. Each of these in-house experts needs additional training in identification and crisis management as well as good working relationships with appropriate community agencies and private therapists.

THE STRUCTURE AND CONTENT OF ASAP

Once a school community conquers the fear and denial that so often prevent schools from implementing a suicide awareness program, the major problem is the method of disseminating this sensitive material to parents, teachers, and students, which often proves an insurmountable stumbling block. As a result, comprehensive programs are infrequently implemented and rarely maintained past the initial phase. Numerous logistical and attitudinal problems must be identified and addressed if the school intends to provide more than a one-shot program.

Each program contains the key information previously outlined. The following are the basic components in the order in which ASAP is most frequently introduced:

1. *Educators' seminar.* This is a two- to three-hour intensive seminar for teachers, administrators, and school support staff. Each program consists of a variety of training strategies, including lectures, audiovisual materials, self-evaluation exercises, small-group discussions, case histories, and role playing. The objectives of these programs are to develop a common understanding of the causes and warning signs of adolescent suicide, teach specific intervention skills, clarify school procedures for handling troubled teenagers, and familiarize educators with specific community agencies and therapists who are available to work with suicidal adolescents.

2. *Parents' program.* This is a flexible educational and awareness program tailored to the needs and interests of the particular group of participants. Programs vary from a thirty-minute overview to an intensive two-hour seminar, but are specially designed to reduce denial and to offer support to concerned parents.

3. *Students' workshop.* This unique four-to-six-hour workshop is designed to provide students in the ninth or tenth grades with accurate, straightforward information about adolescent suicide. In addition to learning key information, students study the developmental stages of adolescence, evaluate their own emotional well-being, practice identifying depression and suicidal behavior, and make recommendations about the actions that local students, schools, parents, and community groups can take to reduce the feelings of alienation and despair in young people.

4. *Primary prevention programs.* These specially tailored programs are developed in cooperation with school personnel once the first three components of ASAP are in place. The mental health center provides initial consultation and, when indicated, staff to begin the programs. These programs are introduced only after the basic ASAP training has been completed and the entire system has been sensitized. Typical programs include student discussion groups, workshops on stress management and communication and relationship skills, and peer counseling programs in which junior and senior students are trained to provide support to troubled classmates.

Although each component has a core curriculum and implementation procedure, individual programs are designed to meet each school system's current or unique situation, such as the recent suicide of a student or faculty member. School personnel may play an active role in implementing each segment. The program uses existing school personnel and is designed to be cost effective and readily replicated.

The educators' seminar and parents' programs are led by specially trained mental health educators from the local mental health center. The students' workshop is initially introduced by the mental health agency staff, but an in-house school team consisting of a range of school personnel is concurrently trained to take over the conduct of the workshops.

The students' workshops are then given annually to each incoming ninth- and tenth-grade class by the school's ASAP team, which usually consists of guidance counselors, members of the child study team, grade-level advisors, and school nurses. The sponsoring mental health agency continues to provide emergency and therapeutic services to troubled teenagers and their families, as well as program consultation to the ASAP team.

Periodic retraining of faculty and parents is required. School staff usually require a refresher course every four to five years and the parents' programs are frequently offered to the families of students currently enrolled in the students' workshop, as well as other concerned community members. A school-based ASAP coordinator is needed to ensure the smooth and timely scheduling of training every year.

The coordinators of the various schools meet twice a year in a group with the mental health center staff to review procedures, view new training films, and learn about new developments in the field of adolescent suicide prevention. These meetings help perpetuate the program, give recognition to the schools' ASAP team, and ensure good working relations and referral procedures between the school and the mental health agency.

EVALUATION

Since the inception of ASAP, approximately 4,700 educators, 3,600 students, and more than 3,000 parents have participated in the program. Each workshop is evaluated with a simple rating scale immediately after the program. Although the participants' scores have been routinely excellent, the long-term impact of the program on attitudes and behavior has not been measured. A thorough and rigorous evaluation of ASAP is now in the planning and funding stages.

The other informal measures of ASAP's impact include the following:

Increase in the number of referrals. We tend to average between three and five referrals from a school system after the introduction of each program element. These youngsters referred tend to be ones who were *not* known to the child study team, but had confided in a classroom teacher or been identified by a support staff member.

Approximately one-quarter to one-third of these referrals become active cases. Many children who are referred are not actively suicidal; rather, they are troubled young people in need of counseling. Students also appear to be more comfortable in referring themselves or a friend for counseling after they have participated in the students' workshop. They also make frequent and more appropriate use of the agency's original emergency service.

Less resistance to asking for help. Parents and teenagers appear less reluctant to accept a referral to the mental health center and are more willing to follow through on treatment recommendations after participating in ASAP.

Improved communications. Contact and communications are strengthened among school staff, especially the administration, the child study team, and the mental health professionals. School and mental health center staff gain a better understanding and appreciation of each other's problems, procedures, and concerns. Referral and feedback difficulties are fewer and more easily resolved when the parties involved know one another.

Enhanced confidence between students and ASAP personnel. As was previously noted, most people are reluctant to discuss suicide with teenagers. Adolescents want and need this life-and-death information and respect the agency staff for talking directly about a taboo subject. Their level of trust and positive attitude toward the program presenters appears to increase after participation.

Decrease in the number of adolescent suicides in Bergen County. The reported number of adolescent suicides has decreased dramatically since the inception of ASAP in 1980. Although we are unable to say that the decrease is a direct result of ASAP, we can identify numerous cases in which a youngster at risk was identified *before* a suicide attempt was made. Clinical experience indicates that we have made many critical interventions with previously undiagnosed teenagers.

ASAP is a flexible curriculum that lends itself to additions and modifications. The staff is currently working on a number of program additions, including these:

- introductory workshops for seventh and eight graders to focus on self-image, communication skills, adolescent development, problem solvings, and stress management;
- refresher seminars for graduating seniors to prepare them for the stresses of separation from high school and entering college or going to work;
- modification of the ASAP curriculum for "survivor schools" (systems that have experienced a student or faculty suicide in the past twelve months);
- exploration of the possibility of involving survivors of suicide in both school and ASAP staff training;
- development of strategies to involve other community systems that work with youngsters — law enforcement personnel, pediatricians, the clergy, hospital and emergency room staff, and funeral directors; and

- implementation of workshops and seminars geared to the concerns of inner-city youths.

CONCLUSIONS

From the initial pilot program in 1980 to the county-wide implementation of ASAP in 1985, we frequently have modified and revised the content and training methodology. Two convictions remain part of our guiding framework:

1. Effective adolescent suicide awareness and prevention education must involve all members of a school community — administrators, educators, parents, and students.
2. To maximize the effectiveness of a suicide prevention program, local school communities and mental health professionals must be joined in a cooperative working partnership.

Both of these convictions are based on eight years of work on the subject, as well as many false starts and wrong turns. We know there is no perfect adolescent suicide awareness and prevention program. Our program can and will be changed and improved. Although our efforts cannot eradicate suicide, we can educate our community the best way we know how.

16

Death Education as a Preventive Approach in Promoting Mental Health

Robert G. Stevenson

Mental health professionals are increasingly coming to accept the definition of bereavement as mourning the loss of something precious, whether it be a person (through death or divorce), a condition (health), a career potential (college rejection), or a feeling (such as self-confidence). Given this definition of bereavement, young students throughout the country deal with loss and bereavement every day.

To help understand the effects of loss, let us look at some statistics. By their senior year in high school, one in twenty children will lose a parent to death. This means that in any given class of students, the odds are that at least one has lost a parent to death. Each year, one in 750 school-age children will die. This means that any school of 1,000 or more students should expect to lose one or more children to death each year. Yet the years when no deaths occur are taken for granted, and when a death does occur, it is almost always treated as a unique event, one that has never happened before and will never happen again.

The reality, of course, is that students lose principals and teachers and learn of the deaths of community members. They must cope with the death of siblings, because more people die in the first year of life than in any of the next forty years. Yet bereaved children are expected to return to the classroom after a short interval and resume business as usual. Far too often, children are disciplined by teachers because their grades have dropped after the death of a sibling. The grief of these children is complicated by the guilt they are made to experience for not maintaining a previously high level of academic performance, when in fact they are performing a great feat just by being in school and functioning at all.

Children also are bereaved by the death of their beloved family pets. Recently, our family cat disappeared. It had been ill and one Friday did not come home at night. For two days we searched, first for the cat and then for the body. My oldest son, Robert, was crushed. On Monday morning, I saw him crying as he combed his hair before going to school. I asked him if he would like to stay home for the day. He nodded yes, and his younger brother stayed home to keep him company. They did not just want a day off from school. They stayed home because my oldest son was suffering through a profound grief experience. If one of our immediate family members had died, I do not think that it could have caused him any more emotional pain than he experienced that first week after Louis, our cat, disappeared. He asked, "Will it ever stop hurting?" and "How can you stand it when it hurts this bad?" I believe that some of his teachers would have been furious had they known that he had missed a day of class over "just" a cat. They would have been unable to understand how that had been a meaningful loss in his life. They are good people, but they just would not understand.

Many teachers still do not understand how grief affects children. They are not aware that grades usually fall after the loss of a loved one, or that the drop may occur years after the loss because children muster their forces to postpone the grief reaction. A ten-year-old whose parent dies may not suffer a drop in grades until the junior year in high school. Unable to cope with this loss, the student may then exhibit behavioral changes or turn to alcohol or drugs to numb the emotional pain. How often do schools stop at the symptom without seeking the real cause—the unresolved earlier loss of a loved one?

After a serious loss has occurred, it is difficult to provide effective interventions. In order to help children prepare to live through the losses they will inevitably encounter, we must take effective action before the loss occurs, not after the fact.

By way of illustration, let us look at the way schools reacted to the 1986 Challenger space shuttle tragedy. In my high school, many educators wanted to do the "right thing," but they themselves were in shock. In fact no one really knew *what* to do and so, other than setting up televisions so that the students could watch the explosion over and over again, no one did anything. There was no general announcement. The entire school observed a moment of silence, which was followed by one teacher's emotional tribute to school teacher-astronaut Christa MacAuliffe. However, not all students identified personally with Christa MacAuliffe, and some were angered by the assumption that they did. They personalized the loss by identifying with someone else in the crew and perceived the failure to mention the other six as a personal slight. Soon thereafter a bulletin was posted to honor the seven, and this dissipated much of these students' anger.

On the second day, the school responded well, but why had it done nothing on that important first day? The school, as does each school in New Jersey, holds two fire drills each month. We have never had a fire in our school, but the fire drills proceed regardless. In contrast, a month does not go by without some students losing loved ones. Scarcely a year goes by without some sort of loss in the community. But we have never, in any significant way, tried to think through an answer to the question of what we can do to help these children when losses occur.

The students in our course "Perspectives on Death" helped us to construct some guidelines for dealing with loss in the school. Teachers and students said that the first thing they remember when facing a loss and wondering what to do was a series of questions, and the guidelines are built around these.

Who should tell the students? This person does not have to be someone with whom the student is close. We suggest that it be someone in authority. By having a principal give the news, we say to the student that his or her loss is important; that is why this person who is important in the school is breaking the news. It is preferable to have the principal rather than the superintendent of schools do so because the principal is part of the daily lives of the students, whereas, in most cases, the superintendent is not.

Someone close to the student (a guidance counselor, another student, a teacher, or the school nurse) should be present and should remain with the student after he or she has been told.

Where should the student be told? It should be a private place where the student can remain and rest after learning the news. In most schools, the nurse's office meets these requirements.

How should the student be told? The person who tells the student should do so in the same manner that he or she would wish to be told. To reassure the person doing the telling, several suggestions can be offered:

- Be simple and direct.
- State what has happened; avoid platitudes and euphemisms.
- Be certain the student really understands what has been said.
- Speak quietly and directly.
- Do not offer unnecessary details, but if the student asks questions, and if you know the answers and are able to respond, then tell exactly what you know as you know it.

What should one do after telling the student? Be aware that students will react in different ways and that some may not react visibly at all. In some cases, the student may wish to return to class and will try to act as though nothing has happened. When one aspect of a person's life is falling apart and seems to be beyond his control, he may try to balance it by having as much control as possible over other areas of his life. One student, for example, wanted to keep statistics at a basketball game the night after his grandmother had died. His parent yelled at him for wanting to "enjoy" himself, but that was not the point. He was trying to meet what he saw as a personal responsibility to show that he still had some control over his life.

After the Challenger shuttle tragedy, some students became upset because they did not "feel" anything at all. They said they knew that a terrible thing had happened, but that they did not feel anything inside. They wanted to know what was "wrong" with them. Thus, an educator must be prepared to support the individual student the way that he or she needs to be supported, not according to some general formula.

Of course, when the loss affects the entire school, other policies are needed. Within ten minutes of the explosion of the Challenger space shuttle, I heard a rumor in my school that Christa MacAuliffe had been speaking to her students at Concord High School when the blast occurred. The story was wrong. It was a misunderstanding of the fact that she had planned to communicate with the students in the high school at several points in the flight. The students could not be said to have been comforted by the correction of the misstatement because the loss was too great, but they were relieved that this terrible scene, at least, had not taken place. These deaths affected every child and every staff member in the school. It was clear that everyone who was affected could not be told individually. It was equally clear that the students had to be told clearly and accurately because rumors at a time like this can have a terrible effect.

To prevent a recurrence of the inertia we felt on the day of the Challenger tragedy, the administrators and teachers in our school have created the following policy for dealing with "community grief."

- A general announcement will be made that all students should remain in their classes and that they will receive more information shortly.
- Students will then be informed in class about what has happened. A principal can do the telling in a small school; a designated team of people can do so in a larger school. Students will be told exactly what happened and their questions answered to try to head off rumors.
- When all classes have been informed, there will be a general announcement to confirm that what they have been told is indeed what has happened. There may be a moment of silence.
- While the teachers are with their classes (after the class-by-class announcement has been made), they can discuss possible memorials, how one behaves during a condolence visit, and possible effects of the loss, or they can simply listen to what the students want to say at this time.

It has been pointed out that it might be better to say nothing to the students, just allow time for personal reflection. However, the avoidance of displays of strong emotion are not necessarily better for the students. The students are aware of how they feel. If we choose to do nothing, then students will reach one of two conclusions: that we adults, whom students see as problem solvers, are not capable of doing anything; or that we could do something to help but instead choose not to do so. Students who reach the first conclusion may decide that if adults, with all of their knowledge and experience, cannot help, then they must be "helpless" as well. Those who reach the second conclusion will believe that we are indifferent. If we choose to do nothing, we are still teaching, but the lessons are helplessness and indifference, both of which are detrimental.

Students who are offered no forum for their thoughts and feelings will still attempt to make them known. After the shuttle disaster, many students resorted to "humor" to try to open up the topic. One week after the incident, my younger son and I discussed the stories about the astronauts he had heard, which were troubling him. Two weeks after the episode, my older son heard the same stories in his high school. This pattern was reported by other teachers and parents; it became clear that many of these stories were starting with younger children and being repeated by older ones. Almost four weeks after the disaster, my students began to chronicle "adult" versions of this shuttle humor. The children's stories dealt with physical disintegration and the decomposition of the bodies — this, their key fear, came up over and over again in the stories. The "humor" of the adults dealt with sports analogies and sex.

If it is true that we joke about what we fear, then these stories were consistent with child development. One junior high school student woke up terrified from a dream that she had found the head of a woman astronaut under her bed. She was just reaching sexual maturity, and bodily integrity was a major issue for her. To hear that the two women astronauts had disintegrated was disturbing to her, but she could not speak about it. Instead she had been telling the story about how people know that one astronaut had dandruff because they found her "head and shoulders." The joke was her attempt to express her concerns, but listeners were so horrified that they just wanted to change the topic and not follow it up with any questions. Finally, her description of her nightmares served to open the topic for the discussion that she had sought with her "humor." If people are unwilling to talk about a problem, a child may try to shock them into doing so.

When nothing else is done at the "teachable moment," should we be startled when children say that they never want their parents to take a "shuttle" flight to Washington or Boston again? For many of these children the actions of the school became a key to developing positive coping mechanisms, a place to "talk about it." Talking about a problem allows us to feel that we have some control over it; silence makes it look as though the problem controls us.

The shuttle disaster was a real test for the schools. When it happened, administrators who already had policies in effect did not have to pause and ask, What should we do now? Fires, severe storms, bomb threats are all crisis situations for which schools have established policies. Surely the pain faced by school children who are dealing with a major loss, individually or collectively, is also a crisis situation. Mental health professionals, school administrators, teachers, and parents must make very effort to assure that we have appropriate policies for that as well.

17

The St. Francis Project:
A Preventive Mental Health Model for Adolescents

William A. Wendt and A. Elaine Cummings

During adolescence, young people finally establish a dominant, positive ego identity, which includes coming to terms with the anxieties and fears associated with death, and all the consequences of understanding mortality. As Erikson (1964) and others have noted, adolescence is a major time of bereavement. In a culture that has denied and avoided the psychosocial issues related to death, however, the problems in coping with the bereavement associated with any separation or loss have received little, if any, attention in the schools.

In its course "Death and Dying: A Course about Life and Living," which is designed as a preventive service, the St. Francis Center in Washington, D.C. addresses the areas of bereavement associated with entering and going through adolescence. On the premise that every separation or loss is a mini-death experience, the curriculum of the course deals not only with the numerous losses in adolescence — the loss of childhood, the loss of innocence, the loss of the sense of a benign world, and the anticipated loss of the comforts of home and family — but also with the difficult experiences of parental separation and divorce, the death of a family member, and the death of a friend or classmate.

The primary goal of death education is to give adolescents a systematic, introspective experience that will help them improve the quality of their lives as they face the unlimited prospects and dangers of society. Never before has this society been more conscious of death and its implications. The growing number of older people, the increase of cancer and AIDS, the increase in suicide among old and young alike, the anxieties associated with horrendous death (linked to the Holocaust, environmental disasters, child abuse, and other senseless tragedies), and the fictional and nonfictional presentations of these themes in the media are all indicators of the preoccupation with death. To a considerable degree, however, the primary social institutions — the church, the family, and the school — have been caught up in the cultural avoidance and denial of death and so have largely abdicated their traditional roles and rituals in helping people come to terms with death.

Today, young people need support for self-development in a too-often hostile world. As Erikson (1964:340) rightly noted, "Youth after youth, bewildered by his assumed role, a role forced on him by the inexorable standardization of American adolescence, are increasingly in danger of losing connection with their dreams, idiosyncracies, roles, and skills." Death education is vital to adolescents' ability to cope with the universal problem of how to come to terms with life and feel some ownership in all that is related to life, including death.

THE ST. FRANCIS PROJECT

After seven years' experience in responding to the requests of schools for support and consultation for school-related deaths, including students' bereavements and suicides; and in the implementation by the St. Francis faculty of death education curricula, the St. Francis Center responded to the dearth of research (Crase and Crase 1984) on the effectiveness of death education for high school students by obtaining grants from two private foundations. The aim of the grants was to do the following: (1) expand the center's educational efforts; (2) make use of psychiatric and educational consultants; and (3) create an assessment effort, in cooperation with a research team from George Washington University, Washington, D.C. The effort involved the participation in a 48-hour curriculum of 120 students from a wide variety of socioeconomic backgrounds who attended six high schools — inner-city and suburban, public and private.

The research protocol was established to examine significant gains in knowledge and changes in attitudes about the issues presented. The evaluation utilized written pre- and post-test instruments, on-site analyses by a project observer, individual and group interviews with students, and a close examination of the students' self-expression assignments.

Findings

It was clear that a high percentage of the students, some of whom were assigned to the course and some of whom selected it, thought they had experienced a significant loss and did not have a sufficient emotional outlet until they participated in this course. It was equally clear that the class experience had strengthened the bonds between students and increased the support systems among peers and between students and the staff. It was important for the students that this experience was school based — that it was "on their own turf."

The students were able to identify and examine loss and separation issues that related to their own stage in life — death of a mother, the murder of a brother, the loss of a girlfriend, failing an important test, or being rejected from a team. An examination of the students' assignments revealed strong and healthy examples of self-expression, problem-solving skills, a clarification of values, and positive philosophies for living. By grappling with the meaning of death and its implications for their lives, the students seemed to emerge with a new maturity and greater emotional health.

CONCLUSIONS

Many suicides by young people are evidently related to unresolved grief (the loss of relationships, of expectations, or of self-respect). Students in the St. Francis project were able to talk about their own past attempts and the related grief, with beneficial results. We believe that a course offering such as ours that teaches students to examine their resolutions, coping skills, and resources can be an effective suicide prevention program. Death education has helped these students to clarify the bewilderment to which Erikson referred and to reconnect with their dreams, roles, and skills. As one 17-year-old boy reported: "It is a chance for us to learn about who we are and what we are about — not just more of what is expected of us."

REFERENCES

Crase, D. R., and D. Crase. 1984. "Death Education in the Schools for Older Children." In H. Wass and C. A. Corr, eds. *Childhood and Death*. New York: Hemisphere Publishing Co.

Erikson, E. 1964. *Childhood and Society*, 2nd ed. New York: W. W. Norton & Co.

PART 3

Illness, Aging, and Bereavement

18

Spontaneous Abortion and Grieving

Jack M. Stack

Many events in the reproductive experience of women and their families include losses. These events include infertility, miscarriage, elective abortion, therapeutic abortion, ectopic pregnancy, stillbirth, prematurity, neonatal injury, neonatal death, birth of a disabled child, and adoption. These experiences have the dynamic characteristics of a loss, but often are not recognized as a loss by caregivers, friends, family members, or even by the women themselves.

Pregnancy and birthing can be viewed as a period of developmental crisis (Bibring et al 1961). The woman and other members of her family begin to develop a relationship with the new baby long before it is born. They have conscious fantasies about what the baby will be like and have good and bad dreams about it. They consider names for it and often give the fetus a temporary nickname.

The new mother will be forever transformed from a separate, self-contained person to a mother with a unique relationship to another person, the baby, who represents itself as a separate person, a part of herself, and a part of another outside love object, the baby's father. In addition, the mother's relationship with her parents, especially her mother, undergoes a major shift when she becomes a mother herself (Friday 1978, Heilbrun 1981).

At the time of birth of a healthy, normal baby, the mother and father usually experience a major release of emotional energy. They say good-bye to their unborn baby and hello to their newborn baby, of a specific sex, whom they see as perfect and unique, and they begin a new phase of attachment to this new person.

When everything goes well with a pregnancy, delivery, and new baby, women and their families may have problems with the tasks of personal growth and attachment. When a casualty occurs, all the members need special care.

One of the most common aspects of reproductive casualties is that they are common and neglected, both in medical practice and in the medical literature. This chapter discusses the range of reproductive losses, from infertility to adoption, reviews the literature on miscarriage, and presents seven case examples of women who have experienced a spontaneous abortion.

THE RANGE OF REPRODUCTIVE LOSSES

Infertility is a major narcissistic blow to both men and women; moreover, the procedures for its diagnosis and treatment have a psychological impact on both men and women. Pregnancy is sometimes a result of individuals' need to prove their fertility and often results in a subsequent elective abortion. Even a wanted or planned pregnancy is accompanied by ambivalence early in the first trimester of pregnancy — the narcissistic stage. The loss of pregnancy in the first trimester by spontaneous miscarriage or ectopic pregnancy is often followed by profound grief, which frequently is ignored by the woman's family and caregivers (Stack 1980, 1984).

The dynamics of the emotional responses to spontaneous abortion, elective abortion, and therapeutic abortion differ. Issues such as planned pregnancy, whether the woman wants to have a baby, the woman's sense of control over events and decisions, the presence of unresolved ambivalence, and a feeling of support from others are important to her ability to deal with the emotional conflict that is inherent in these major decisions and losses.

Stillbirth, the birth of a dead baby after the twentieth week, is a major loss for the woman and her family. However, it is rarely treated as such by the caregivers or society. Similarly, the birth of an injured, deformed or premature baby is an assault upon a woman's self-image and expectations and jeopardizes her ability to bond to and care for the baby. Even the death of a newborn is often not recognized as a major loss by family and friends. Incomplete or pathological grief syndromes can develop with these losses and may interfere with the woman's ability to care for her other or subsequent children.

Birth mothers who give up their babies for adoption rarely have adequate counseling and are often left with broken hearts and anniversary grief reactions; years later, they will often search for the child, either in their fantasies or in reality (Colon 1973; Lifton 1978; Sorosky, Baran, and Pannor 1984; Stack 1979, 1981).

Spontaneous Abortion

Miscarriage and its management can serve as a prototype to illustrate the nature of these losses and the responses of caregivers. Spontaneous abortion is a loss experienced at a personal and intrapsychic level to a much greater degree than is recognized by family members and friends, or even by the woman herself at a conscious level. The woman is subject to a grieving process and is vulnerable to pathological or unresolved grief reactions.

Many physicians do not acknowledge the existence of grief following a miscarriage. Although they recognize that women do tend to feel attached to the fetus during pregnancy, they generally assume that this attachment does not begin until after quickening, when the mother begins to identify with the fetus as a separate person.

Spontaneous abortion is the termination by natural causes of a pre-viable pregnancy. The majority of spontaneous abortions occur in the first trimester of pregnancy, when the woman experiences the developing fetus as an integral part of herself. Nearly 10 percent of all pregnancies end in spontaneous abortion of random and nonrecurring causes. Unresolved, incomplete, and pathological grief reactions are common complications of spontaneous abortion.

REVIEW OF THE LITERATURE

A review of the literature reveals that little attention has been given to the psychological effects of spontaneous abortion, although there has been some discussion of the psychological factors in habitual abortion, and of the benefits of psychotherapy to assist habitual aborters to carry a baby to term. Many obstetricians observe a higher incidence of a second spontaneous abortion in the six months following a miscarriage, but the link has not been made between this observation and the fact that six months is often the normal grief period.

In their study of one hundred couples who experienced an early miscarriage or later stillbirth or neonatal death Peppers and Knapp (1980) found no difference in intensity of maternal mourning in relation to the gestational age at which the loss occurred. Horowitz (1979) observed that some teenagers whose pregnancies ended in miscarriage tried to relieve the grief and mourning by becoming pregnant again soon.

Kaij and colleagues (1969) observed evidence of poor postpartum mental health in women with a history of spontaneous abortion and noted that the subjects who had undergone a spontaneous abortion were more likely than the control patients to have lost a father and suffered early neurotic symptoms combined with bereavement. The authors hypothesized that there are psychological influences on spontaneous abortion. They suggested that an unsuccessful identification with the mother is a common factor among women with a history of miscarriage. The mothers of women in this group were described as possessive, dominating, punitive, and intolerant; the fathers were absent, dead, or detached. But although the authors focused on the causation of miscarriage in terms of bereavement, absence or loss of a father, and symptoms of neurosis, they failed to respond to their original observation: the evidence of emotional disorder among women with a history of spontaneous abortion. It is possible that a higher incidence of previous unresolved loss, as well as incomplete grieving for the miscarriage itself, may have contributed to the women's poor mental health.

There is evidence that some women do not completely resolve their grief following a miscarriage. Peppers and Knapp (1980) described a "shadow grief" ranging from eight to twenty years after a miscarriage, and Stack (1980) reported the persistence of unresolved grief with flooding of emotion during subsequent interviews ten to twenty-one years after a miscarriage. Corney and colleagues (1974) described a case of pathological grief following miscarriage and observed that this grief reaction was not fully addressed in the literature. Stack (1980) also reported a case of delayed grief reaction resulting in organic illness that was resolved only after an intensive working through of the loss.

Simon and colleagues (1969) compared thirty-two women who had miscarried with forty-six women who had had therapeutic abortions, primarily for psychiatric reasons. Although none of the women in the miscarriage group had a previous history of psychiatric illness, thirteen in that group reported depressed feelings at the time of the miscarriage and eight had a subsequent diagnosis of psychiatric illness. The authors reported that no psychiatric symptomatology occurred after the therapeutic abortions that were attributale to the abortion. (It is interesting to note that the miscarriage patients were the control group.)

Deutsch (1947) observed that psychogenic factors were clearly responsible for many of the spontaneous abortions she studied. She did not, however, discuss the psychological sequelae of spontaneous miscarriage.

Many case histories of miscarriage and the emotional responses of both men and women have been reported in the literature (Deutsch 1947, Dunbar 1963, Horowitz 1979, Pepper and Knapp 1980, Stack 1980). Although these authors disagree about psychological factors causing miscarriage, they agree that the emotional response can be psychologically devastating. Such descriptors as uncertainty, powerlessness, helplessness, guilt, sadness, disbelief, anger, frustration, blame, and disappointment recur throughout these writings.

Novelists, poets, and biographers, as well as experts on women's issues, have documented the devastating effects of miscarriage (Boston Women's Health Book Collective 1979, Mitchell 1936, Parkes 1972, Stack 1982, Stone 1975, Parkes 1972). In the novel *Gone With The Wind,* Mitchell (1936) extensively described the emotional and physical effects of a miscarriage on the character Scarlett O'Hara. Stone (1975) described the effect of miscarriage on Henry and Sophia Schliemann, the nineteenth-century discoverers of Troy, and related Sophia's flooding of emotion at a later time when she encountered an ancient fetal skeleton in her exploration of a burial urn. In everyday clinical practice, physicians, psychologists, and social workers will find unresolved emotional sequelae of miscarriages when they take detailed reproductive histories.

DISCUSSION

The normal grieving process has been well studied and described (Clayton et al 1974, Lindemann 1944, Parkes 1972). Characteristics of the grieving person include (1) somatic distress, (2) preoccupation with the image of the lost person, (3) guilt feelings, (4) anger and hostility, and (5) changes in normal conduct. Most people who experience a loss, even the death of a spouse, do not see a psychotherapist (Clayton et al 1974). The focus of the mourning process can be normal object loss, such as the death of spouse, parent, or child or the loss of a job — which is recognized as such by the affected individual and by others — or it can be less obvious, such as the loss of spouse by divorce; the loss of self-esteem, appearance, body image, or status; or the death of an unborn child.

If the loss is acknowledged by the person and others, the normal process of mourning can and usually does take place. Caregivers, friends, and loved ones give permission for the grieving person to experience and express a sense of loss. One is allowed to assume a dependent role — to cry, to be held, and to be cared for. Following a period of relative decompensation and disorganization, resolution and restitution usually occur.

Kennell and Klaus (1976) outlined recommendations for helping parents of an infant who has died, whether it was stillborn or died soon after birth. They recommended that the parents be allowed to see and handle the infant and that they have a funeral, avoid using tranquilizers, refrain from having another baby until the mourning reaction is complete, meet with another parent who has lost a baby or with a group of bereaved parents, and that they include their other children in the discussion and understanding of the loss.

Relatives, friends, and even professional caregivers often fail to respond to parents who have had the seemingly obvious loss of a stillborn or a neonate. In the case of a spontaneous abortion, an adequate and helpful response is even less common. Many factors that are unique to this loss explain the development of delayed or pathological grief reactions:

- Frequently, other people do not even know that the woman was pregnant.
- A woman who has miscarried is often embarrassed or reticent about mentioning that she was but is no longer pregnant.
- Frequently the woman had not resolved the ambivalence typical of the early, narcissistic stage of pregnancy.
- She had not identified the fetus as a new person who was also a part of herself. Grieving the loss of one's self is often different from and more difficult than grieving the loss of an outside love object.
- She is unable to identify with the "lost person" even to the extent of having felt fetal movement and recognized that "someone else" was there.
- There is no funeral.
- The woman rarely sees what she has lost.
- Caregivers, family members, and friends often encourage denial and intellectualization with phrases such as "You didn't get to know it," "It was God's will," "It would have been deformed anyway." They rarely encourage the woman to cry, to talk about her loss, and to assume the role of a bereaved person.
- A miscarriage is usually sudden and does not allow the woman a period of anticipatory grieving and preparation for the loss.

- Guilt is a nearly universal feeling among women suffering from a miscarriage. Because explanations of the cause are often inadequate or nonexistent, the woman is led to feel that she may have done something to cause the miscarriage.
- There is a sense of helplessness that occurs when the woman is bleeding and having cramps and neither she nor her physician can do anything to stop the process. As Seiligman (1972) demonstrated experimentally, helplessness is often a cause of despair and depression.

Indications of unresolved grief reactions include: (1) a vivid, clear memory of events surrounding the loss, (2) frequent flashing of the events of that day or of specific scenes of the loss, (3) an anniversary reaction, (4) the persistence of affect such as sadness or anger when talking about the loss, and (5) a flooding of emotion at the time of a subsequent crisis.

CASE REPORTS

Case 1

Carol, a thirty-year-old Catholic registered nurse and mother of two, complained of fatigue, being more susceptible to illnesses such as gastrointestinal upsets, and having a cold that persisted for six weeks. She had expressed anger toward her physician, who had treated her with penicillin, reported a negative chest radiograph, and told her she was neurotic. During the history taking, it emerged that she had had these general symptoms for about four months, ever since an early miscarriage. Further examination revealed a purulent nasal discharge, a labile affect, and a positive radiograph for maxillary sinusitis.

After outlining a program for treating her "real" sinusitis, the therapist said, "Now tell me how you feel about your miscarriage." Carol immediately began to describe, with stark clarity, details of the day of the miscarriage, especially her early denial of the possibility that she was having a miscarriage. Although she had a relative infertility problem and wanted to be pregnant, she acknowledged ambivalence about the pregnancy and the effect that another child would have on her career. Following the miscarriage, she had received little or no emotional support from her physician, her priest, her husband, or her nurse-friend who assisted with her surgical care in the emergency room. She avoided attempts by her parents, her sister, and her supervisor to comfort her because she did not want to burden them (her father had cancer, her sister was in another state, and her supervisor was having marital problems).

Although Carol continued to function with her family and professionally, she did so with great fatigue and increasing resentment and anger. She acknowledged an unfulfilled need to be held, loved, comforted, and allowed to assume the role of a grieving person.

Carol was seen in therapy for four weeks, during which she did significant grief work in therapy sessions and with her family and friends. On sharing her experience with her mother-in-law she found tht her mother-in-law remembered every detail of her own miscarriage, which had occurred twenty years before.

As Carol proceeded through the grief work, her anger subsided, her affect became less labile, the details of the memory of the miscarriage began to blur, and she could talk about her experience without pain. Her chronic fatigue and susceptibility to illness resolved, as did her sinusitis.

Case 2

One of the dynamics of unresolved grief is that the burden becomes a source of interference in some future crisis, flooding the person with old, unresolved emotions. Such was the case with Ann, the fifty-two-year-old registered nurse who had assisted Carol at the time of her treatment in the emergency room. Ten years before, Ann had spontaneously aborted an eighteen-week-old fetus at home. She thought that she had resolved the early ambivalence about the pregnancy and said that her husband and other children had comforted her and cried with her at the time of the miscarriage.

Although Ann acknowledged a feeling of having come closer to her husband and children, she clearly showed evidence of unresolved grief. She recalled that at six months after the miscarriage, the event was still vivid and painful, and that each year she thought about the son who might have been and how old he would be. She ackowledged with tears that she had turned away from her friend in the emergency room because she was flooded with the painful memory of her own miscarriage. We found the following hint of why she had not completed her own grief work: one week after her miscarriage, her oldest daughter was to be married. Ann had stopped her own grief work to care for her daughter; she pulled herself together, "forgot about her own problem," and helped prepare for her daughter's wedding.

Case 3

Mary, a fifty-year-old teacher, had had a miscarriage during her first pregnancy, approximately twenty years before her interview. During the interview, it became clear that the anxiety attacks and the headaches she was suffering from now were a recurrence of symptoms she had first experienced following her miscarriage.

At the time of the miscarriage, Mary and her husband had been entertaining friends. She had received no comforting from her husband or her friends after the miscarriage, and her mother had told her, "I don't know what's wrong with you. I never had that kind of problem." Mary experienced tension headaches and anxiety attacks for approximately two years after the miscarriage without identifying the source of the difficulty. The recurrence of the symptoms at this time followed a hysterectomy, when her mother made a similar comment ("I don't know what's wrong with you.") When discussing the miscarriage, Mary noted details of the events surrounding it with great clarity.

Case 4

Ginny, a thirty-eight-year-old, in discussing her miscarriage of ten years before, noted that when she had begun spotting, her doctor told her, "You're trying to have a miscarriage." Her denial was evident both by her statement, "I am not," and her further behavior. She did not go to bed as instructed, but rather stayed up to iron clean shirts for her husband in case she had to go to the hospital. In the hospital, she bled for three more days and required transfusions before she would allow a dilation and curettage. After that procedure, she complained of a pain in her throat and expressed the fear that she might have throat cancer. Finally, her doctor told her she was having a neurotic reaction and to pull herself together. Her husband told her not to talk about the miscarriage because talking about it would not help. When she spoke with me, she could remember every detail of the days surrounding the miscarriage and experienced strong affect that she identified as anger. When asked if she knew why she was angry, she replied "Yes, because of feeling unable to do anything about it, of being helpless to control the bleeding and the miscarriage."

Case 5

Ellen, a 50-year-old psychologist, had had a spontaneous miscarriage twenty-one years before. She stated that she had grieved, cried, and felt pain, loneliness, loss, despair, guilt, and anger. Initially, it seemed to her and to me that she had completed the grief process. When she filled out a questionnaire about the miscarriage, however, she realized how long the grief process had taken and how incomplete it had really been.

Ellen said that she was angry with both her husband and her doctor for the casual way they had treated her loss at that time. Her attempt to express her feelings to her parents was blocked by their disapproval of her pregnancy and her husband and by their relief that she was not going to have another child. Ellen had talked with her husband without feeling understood or supported. She acknowledged that she felt a sense of loss:

> It was a great loss, but not easily understood, of profound meaning to me, regarding life and death. I had a profound sense that an unknown person and some part of my person had died. It was incredibly confusing and it was treated in a casual manner by others, leaving me with a sense of bewilderment and self-doubt. Yes, I grieve; I wept and felt sad, lonely, and depressed, but it was not a satisfactory grief because it was in isolation. It was not shared with others.

At the time, Ellen wrote a letter to an aunt who had had a miscarriage, hoping to communicate with someone who had endured a similar experience. This is a common response by women who feel a sense of isolation. They feel that no one else has had a similar experience and that there is something wrong with them. Her aunt never answered her letter.

When responding to the questionnaire, Ellen again experienced intense feelings. She remembered that after the birth of her next child, she cried uncontrollably. "People kept asking me what was the matter, but I did not know then." Two years after her miscarriage, a friend delivered a stillborn baby. "I remember that I again cried a great deal for several days, feeling a sense of great loss. I did not know then, but now, as I have answered the questionnaire, I have recalled and associated these experiences with my miscarriage." This case demonstrates isolation, incomplete grieving, and flooding with affect at a later time of crisis.

The following two cases illustrate that women grieve the loss of their babies by miscarriage whether their pregnancy was planned or unplanned, and that women can complete their grieving with their family and friends without, and sometimes in spite of, the caregivers.

Case 6

Linda, a thirty-year-old mother of three, became pregnant even though she had an intrauterine device in place. Although she and her husband were surprised, they wanted another child and readily accepted the pregnancy; then she suffered a spontaneous miscarriage. When Linda was interviewed five years later, she recalled a profound grief reaction, which she had clearly completed with family and friends, especially one friend who had had a similar experience a few years before.

In her responses to the questionnaire, she described one of the behaviors that tend to block grieving. Some people, especially doctors and nurses, make comments such as, "It's for the best," "Try not to think about it," and "Don't be upset; it wasn't a planned pregnancy." She received the impression from the nurses that it really did not matter, since miscarriages are routine non-events for most medical personnel.

Case 7

Beverly, a forty-year-old woman, had miscarried ten years before at the eighth week of gestation. Because she was taking birth control pills at the time, she had not realized that she was pregnant. During the interview, she recalled no early feelings other than being shocked to learn that she was pregnant. She began to have problems when she returned home. "I cried a lot and lost ten pounds in about two weeks." She returned to me (her physician) complaining of dysphoria, fatigue, and other symptoms. I checked her pelvis and hematocrit and told her she was all right. This seems to be the usual pattern; the physician examines the woman and says, "You're O.K.," rather than saying, "How are you? How do you feel about your miscarriage? Do you feel a sense of loss? Are there tears? Are there any words to go with the tears?" Fortunately, Beverly resolved her grief with her family and friends and later was able to be a support person for her friend, Linda. Both of these women, five and ten years later, were able to remember without pain the great sense of loss they had experienced and the inexplicable nature of the loss, "almost to the point of being unable to describe it." Both women clearly felt the need to have another baby and did so. They acknowledged the healing effect of having the subsequent baby. One might speculate that these "makeup babies" were part of the final resolution of their grief.

CONCLUSION

The primary responsibility for the facilitation of normal grieving and for the prevention and detection of delayed, unresolved, and pathological grief reactions rests with the obstetrician and family physician. However, psychiatrists, psychologists, nurses, clergy, and social workers should also be aware of the relatively common occurrence of this syndrome, should assist primary physicians in understanding its dynamics, and should be prepared to search for and treat the unresolved grief. As with other losses, it is important to distinguish these syndromes of inadequate grieving from depression, since treatment techniques, the course of the illness, and the prognosis are often different (Lindemann 1944, Stack 1982).

REFERENCES

Bibring, G. L., T. F. Dwyer, D. S. Huntington, et al. 1961. "Study of the Psychological Processes in Pregnancy and of the Earliest Mother-Child Relationship: Some Propositions and Comments." *Psychoanalytic Study of the Child* 16:19–27.

Boston Women's Health Book Collective. 1979 *Our Bodies, Ourselves,* 2nd ed. New York: Simon & Schuster.

Clayton, P. et al. 1974. "Pathological Grief Following Spontaneous Abortion." *American Journal of Psychiatry* 131:7.

Colon, F. 1973. "In Search of One's Past: An Identity Trip." *Family Practice* 12:429–438.

Corney, R. et al. 1969. "Psychological Grief Following Spontaneous Abortion." *American Journal of Psychiatry* 131:53–59.

Deutsch, H. 1947. *The Psychology of Women,* vol. 2: *Motherhood.* New York: Grune & Stratton.

Dunbar, F. 1963. "Emotional Factors in Spontaneous Abortion." In W. Kroger, ed. *Psychosomatic Gynecology, Obstetrics and Endocrinology.* Springfield IL: Charles C. Thomas.

Friday, N. 1978. *My Mother, My Self. The Daughter's Search for Identity.* New York: Dell Publishing Co.

Heilbrun, C. 1981. *Reinventing Womanhood.* New York: W. W. Norton & Co.

Horowitz, N. 1979. "Adolescent Mourning Reaction to Infant and Fetal Loss." *Social Casework* 59(12):2112–2114.

Kaij, L. et al. 1969. "Psychiatric Aspects of Spontaneous Abortion, II: The Importance of Bereavement, Attachment and Neurosis in Early Life." *Journal of Psychosomatic Research* 13:53–59.

Klaus, M. and J. Kennell. 1976. *Maternal-Infant Bonding.* St. Louis: C. V. Mosby Co.

Lifton, R. J. 1978. *Lost and Found.* New York: Holt, Rinehart & Winston.

Lindemann, E. 1944. "Symptomatology and Management of Acute Grief." *American Journal of Psychiatry* 101:141.

Mitchell, M. 1936. *Gone With the Wind.* New York: Macmillan Co.

Parkes, C. 1972. *Bereavement, Studies in Grief in Adult Life.* New York: International Universities Press.

Peppers, L. and R. Knapp. 1980. *Motherhood and Mourning: Perinatal Death.* New York: Praeger Publishers.

Seiligman, M. 1972. "Learned Helplessness." *American Review of Medicine* 23:407.

Simon, et al 1969. "Psychological Factors Related to Spontaneous and Therapeutic Abortion." *American Journal of Obstetrics and Gynecology* 104:799–808.

Sorosky, A. D., A. Baran, and R. Pannor. 1984. *The Adoption Triangle, The Effects of Sealed Records on Adoptees, Birth Parents, and Adoptive Parents,* 2nd ed. Garden City NY: Doubleday Anchor Press.

Stack, J. M. 1979. "Birth Mothers." Paper presented at Research Day II, Michigan State University, November 1.

Stack, J. M. 1980. "Spontaneous Abortion and Grieving." *American Family Physician* 21(5):99–102.

Stack, J. M. 1981. "Oedipus Was an Adopted Child." Paper presented at the Annual Meeting of the American Orthopsychiatric Assocation.

Stack, J. M. 1982a. "Grief Reactions and Depression in Family Practice: Differential Diagnosis and Treatment." *Journal of Family Practice* 14(2):271–275.

Stack, J. M. 1982b. "Reproductive Casualties: Effects on Families and Professional Caregivers." In L. R. Martin and T. E. Davis, eds. *Seminars in Family Medicine.* New York: Grune & Stratton, pp. 98–104.

Stack, J. M. 1984. "The Psychodynamics of Spontaneous Abortion." *American Journal of Orthopsychiatry* 54(1).

Stone, I. 1975. *The Greek Treasure.* Garden City NY: Doubleday & Co.

19

Psychological Support for Residents of a Women's Shelter Following Sudden Infant Death

Alice L. Cullinan

"Alice—we need you: there's been a tragedy." the phone message was from Terry, the director of a woman's shelter in our upstate New York city. The tone of urgency was unusual for her. "Patrick is dead and I'm afraid how the women are going to react." I did not know who Patrick was, but quickly learned, and recognized a need for crisis intervention. I am a psychologist specializing in thanatology, and frequently am involved in such situations.

Soon thereafter, I arrived at the house, which stands in the city's poor inner district. Terry met me at the door and told me the full story. One of the residents, whom I shall call Pam, had lived and worked there for about five months as she tried to get her life back together. Patrick, her son, had been born shortly after she came to the residence. A happy, continually smiling baby, Patrick seemed to most of these troubled women like a bright beacon, a sign of hope for the future. Rarely did an infant receive more T.L.C. than he, and since his birth the rise in spirit of everyone who lived and worked at the shelter was apparent.

That morning, about 7 A.M., Pam had discovered that her child's body was cold and motionless. The ambulance was called. Within four minutes, paramedics arrived. After attempting cardiopulmonary resuscitation without success, they took the child's body to the hospital. Pam and two other women ran after the ambulance for several blocks to the hospital, unaware that the baby was dead. The next thing Pam knew, she was being interviewed by the police, who wanted to rule out foul play. She still had not been told her baby had died. Pam was black, poor, had had a drinking problem in the past, and was not married. Although there had never been any indications of child abuse with her three other children, the suspicions of the police were aroused, and so the interrogation continued for about forty minutes. Only then did a nurse tell Pam that Patrick had died.

The police brought Pam back to the shelter. It was than about 9:00 A.M.

and many of the residents were gathered in the basement dining room having breakfast. Pam did not join them, but went instead up to the third floor dorm where she and Patrick had slept. It was there that she was found two hours later, hugging the mattress where he had lain and died, a SIDS death (as it later was ruled). When the residents learned of Patrick's death, they reacted in a way typical of people alienated from society, impoverished materially and emotionally, and bereft of the ability to nurture and be nurtured socially. They withdrew into their own private worlds, there to be preoccupied with the painful memories of their losses. Because the director of the shelter had recently learned that she and her husband could not have children, she was unconsciously grieving her loss and felt unable to minister effectively to the needs of the others in their grief.

Many of the residents knew me, for I am called to the shelter occasionally to assist women experiencing emotional trauma. Terry told them I was there to help them *all* and would be in the living room. One by one, the women came in. Many had obviously been crying. There was no talking, and most stared at the floor. The last to enter was Pam herself. I knew that I had first to share my feelings, hoping to model for the women what they could do. I arose and went to the door and hugged her, saying "I'm so sorry. . .it must be awful." "Thank you, it is," was her response. I then asked if any of the other thirteen women present wanted to say or indicate anything to Pam.

Initially the women demonstrated a reserve bordering on paralysis. I realized that they needed "permission" to show their feelings before the group, so I shared my belief that it must awfully hard not only for Pam, but for each of them, because they loved Patrick so much and because losing him might also remind them of other losses. "Yeah, that's right—but what good's talking about it with everybody gonna do?" muttered Elsie, who had known her share of losses. I replied that it sounded as if she had not experienced "feeling the good that can come when somebody else knows the pain you are feeling inside." A tear flowed down her cheek. I asked Ruth, who was sitting next to her, to hold her hand, which she did. After a few minutes, Elsie said "It's not fair. We all loved him so much and he never hurt anybody and. . ." She could not complete the sentence, so I said: "I loved him and I'm mad." "Yeah, but who can you get mad at—God?" "He can take it," I replied. Pam then started talking about her "mad," and added how guilty she felt because she had always been taught to "accept God's will. . .and besides, we gotta be strong and not sissies."

"Says who?" I replied, and there was some laughter. The women began to verbalize their anger, sadness, beliefs, pain, and eventually, past experiences with loss. Finally, someone spoke of her belief in a meaning Patrick's death could have for all of them. It was Maria, an eighteen-year-old who had escaped to the shelter from an abusive husband, who said: "If Patrick brought us closer and gave us love while he lived, why can't his death do the same. . .aren't we closer already?"

As I write, it has been three months since Patrick died. This week I met with Terry, the shelter's director. She told me that she believed that the women's experience of being able to grieve with and support one another, beginning that night and continuing over subsequent weeks and months, had very positive repercussions. "We have continued meeting, sharing now not so much about Parick's loss, but about other losses. We learned from you that it was all right to show feelings, and that we *could* help each other. Nobody flipped out like I though they might, and no one has gotten sick. We're so much closer. . . . to think of the bad effect it could have had on so many. . . ."

The intervention in this crisis, which could occur only because my specialty was known and because I was available, is one of many in which I have participated over the years. Usually my role is to acknowledge the loss verbally and to impart to those who are grief-sricken an awareness of the importance of acknowledging the loss and accompanying feelings. I then speak of the positive consequences that can develop out of a willingness to receive support from others. Once the individual or group learns to grieve, further professional intervention is not usually needed: the process continues on its own. Occasionally, while doing crisis intervention, one can recognize an individual who needs or can benefit from additional professional help. I will take that person aside, gently share any pertinent observations, and give him or her several referrals to choose among.

If no such intervention is available to an individual, family, or group which needs it, denial and blocked grieving can result, to the detriment of short-term and even long-term quality of physical and emotional health. Relationships can become strained and deteriorate; entire families can suffer. In my professional practice, I frequently encounter individuals, couples and families who come for counseling because of problems seemingly unrelated to unresolved grief. We often discover that this "not crying good and loud enough and then being able to smile afterwards" (as one six-year-old boy put it) has resulted in such dynamics as repressed anger and hidden guilt that becomes misplaced into others, as well as overcompensatory behavior that attempts to fill the emptiness precipitated by the loss. Sometimes problem drinking develops, as does physical illness. Children who feel isolated and abandoned in their grief and trauma are likely to experience social problems and difficulties in school.

Prevention through appropriate intervention by professionals or paraprofessionals trained in techniques of crisis and bereavement counseling is a task that in earlier eras was done by the family, the neighborhood and the church. The oft-remarked erosion of these institutions has created a void. Today, in many social systems, it is thought inappropriate to grieve openly or express negative feelings. Tranquilizers are often administered instead of hugs. "Being strong" seems to substitute for "It must hurt so much. How can I (we) help?" Consequently there is a serious need for greater use of intervention geared toward prevention in the area of bereavement counseling. More professionals and paraprofessionals should be trained so that when tragedies occur—not only on a global scale, but within marital, family and group systems—intervention can be made available.

20

Scoliosis, Loss, and Grief: A Study in Preventive Mental Health

Frances K. Forstenzer and David P. Roye

In our view it is self-evident that the most effective preventive mental-health approach for adolescents with scoliosis involves understanding and anticipating the possible responses of both the family and the patient. This chapter looks briefly at ideas pertaining to a sense of loss; initial responses of sadness, numbness, or anger; the level of trauma or chronicity; and various emotional styles of handling the diagnosis and treatment of scoliosis. The more thoroughly the implications for the adolescent and her family are understood, the more successful will be the identification of at-risk patients. Consequently, dangers to the patient's psychological equilibrium may be anticipated and treated preventively.

The ideas discussed in this chapter were generated as part of the Forstenzer-Roye Study of Psychosocial Sequelae of Scoliosis in Adolescents. Data were gathered through two interviews of adolescent girls, one year apart, and questionnaires filled out by parents on both occasions. This study is a longitudinal survey. At the time of writing, sixty adolescents have been involved; the study is scheduled to continue until 150 adolescents have been interviewed.

EMOTIONAL RESPONSES TO A DIAGNOSIS

With scoliosis, as with any chronic-disease diagnosis, issues of loss and grief have to be addressed and worked through. Although loss can take many forms, in this context it refers to the patient's sense of having lost the feeling of being "whole" or "perfect," with all parts correctly assembled and in working order. For the parents, the loss is that of the imagined "perfect" child. In scoliosis, the loss is predominantly one of self-image, since there is no real loss of function. Other chronic conditions may involve loss in both areas and are therefore more complicated.

For both the patient and parents, the experience of loss is reflected in a diminished sense of self. The initial response to the diagnosis is often acute and painful. It may be followed by waves of sadness and anger, which parents in the scoliosis project have described as an occurrence both for themselves and for their daughters. The girls have described an initial period of numbness and confusion during which they try to evaluate their parents' response. Much of their own reaction seems to be in relation to what they sense in their parents, in the same way that they have learned their general coping styles at home.

The overall traumatic impact of the diagnosis seems to be affected by what is occurring in the family at the time of the diagnosis. Obviously, overburdened families who are already dealing with excessive stress will be further stressed by having to deal with a medical problem. It is interesting to note, however, that families for whom things are going well often seem to be more seriously thrown off balance, perhaps because effective coping strategies are not in place. Clearly the traumatic impact of such a diagnosis can be assessed and understood only by determining the meaning of the diagnosis within each family system, rather than by merely assessing the level of stress manifest in the family.

Dealing with emergencies requires a different level of psychological energy than does dealing with a chronic, long-term diagnosis of any kind. A scoliosis patient can look forward to the end of the bracing period or to the completion of surgery, but possession of the diagnosis goes on for life. In other kinds of chronic disease (juvenile diabetes, for example) the ongoing and serious nature of the diagnosis requires adaptation to chronicity in intrapsychic terms as well as in terms of concrete medical management.

ADAPTIVE AND MALADAPTIVE RESPONSES

As with all psychological functioning, different youngsters deal with grief and loss according to their past experiences. One unsuccessful style of coping is denial, usually with some breakthrough feelings of discomfort that are not consciously tied to the loss.

Sometimes denial is blatant, as revealed by the following dialogue with Gina, aged thirteen.

> *Interviewer:* When were you first diagnosed as having scoliosis?
>   *Gina:* I don't have scoliosis.
> *Interviewer:* Then why are you here?
>   *Gina:* I have a little problem with my shoulder.
> *Interviewer:* Can you tell me a little bit about your problem?
>   *Gina:* Not really, but it's not scoliosis. It will go away soon.

In all other areas, Gina was functional and able to identify and deal with reality. In this area, she was clearly using denial as a defense. The threat to the organization of her psychological functioning had to be severe, because her attempt to defend was not subtle and because she made no attempt to integrate into her reality the information that was clearly given to her by her parents and the doctor. In addition to the obvious psychological danger to her, it is likely that the extent of her compliance with the physician's directions will be unpredictable.

A less blatant kind of denial is shown in the girls' responses to the question "Since you can't see or feel this scoliosis, do you ever wonder if it is really there?" More than 50 percent of the sixty girls questioned replied that they did wonder or that they realized it must be there but wondered if it really mattered. Considering that the girls are given an opportunity to look at their radiographs, this response is significant. It indicates partial denial, which also serves a defensive purpose but, since the defense is less dramatic, they are more likely than Gina to comply with the physician's directions.

Another unsuccessful way of dealing with loss and grief is to exhibit a significant amount of anger. Often anger is manifest in refusals to comply with treatment. Girls who will not wear a brace or do exercises and consistently fail to keep appointments demonstrate their angry resistance and seem to be inviting adults to be angry at them so that a battle can ensue. This battle over compliance then provides a means for them to express their heretofore unexpressed anger over the initial narcissistic injury. In some instances, magical thinking is involved. The adolescent feels, "I don't really need that brace. It'll be O.K. anyway. I know and the adults don't know." Sometimes this behavior is part of an overall oppositional behavior pattern in which the youngster is essentially saying "I won't because I'm supposed to or because you, the adult, want me to."

A more successful adaptation to loss and grief is shown by adolescents who are able to work through their anger and sadness by talking and crying, and who successfully reorganize their self-concept, using both family and professional support as needed. The diagnosis (whether it be scoliosis or any other chronic condition) is then assigned a more moderate role within the context of the adolescent's life, so that school, friends, and achievements again occupy center stage. Compliance is no problem with this group of patients.

Another relatively successful adaptation involves some ability to talk through emotional responses and a partial, negotiated ability to comply. For example, a sixteen-year-old girl who had been wearing a brace for two years reported, "I just can't wear it to school any more. All last year, I promised myself that it I could get through the year, that would be it. But I can wear it after school and at night. Can we make a deal?" Further exploration of this girl's feelings revealed a real desire to negotiate so that her scoliosis would be treated, and to have the emotional urgency of her feeling about the brace recognized.

Another way of experiencing loss and grief involves defensive isolation of affect. Essentially, the painful affect is successfully blocked out but not denied, in that it can be reached through questioning, dealt with briefly, and then replaced in isolation. Although this is not the most desirable style, it is effective in allowing the youngster to move ahead with the tasks of adolescence. The pressure-cooker effect of denial is avoided, since the feelings are experienced and, to some extent, worked through.

As with family systems, the individual's sense of loss and handling of grief needs to be assessed. One of the factors that needs to be taken into account is that of the adolescent's usual coping mechanisms, as opposed to new defenses that seem to have been activated in response to the diagnosis. For example, a mother reported that her daughter generally talked openly about her worries and concerns but was unwilling to talk about her scoliosis or her brace. This need to alter familiar coping styles may be a signal that the threat is more than the usual mechanisms can handle and that help is needed.

Another factor that has to be considered is the question of who owns the feelings being expressed. Frequently, the girls who have been interviewed have seen the scoliosis as being less threatening than have their parents. In this situation, they pick up and express their parents' anxieties although their own feelings are not so acute. Thus, it is useful to help families and patients understand the source of the feelings, and to recognize that each family member is truly free to have his or her own feelings and to talk about them without being concerned that the feelings may not be acceptable.

Finally, it is important to respect and give credence to the adolescents' feelings and thoughts without jumping in too quickly to deny the significance and reality of these feelings. Adults may often be in a hurry to offer comfort without realizing that the suffering adolescent has intense feelings. Although scoliosis is not a serious illness, the sense of loss is often acute for a time, and grieving over this loss is a necessary process that should be encouraged.

In summary, the best preventive measure for mental health is knowledge that can then be used to build protective services into the existing system of medical care. This kind of knowledge is best gathered by listening attentively to the adolescents and their families whose life experiences we are trying to understand.

21

Family Reactions to Chronic Mental Illness

Francine Cournos

Families mourn the loss of a child to the ravages of chronic mental illness like they do the loss of child who dies (Walsh 1985). This chapter examines some of the reasons for grief among families of the severely mentally ill and the ways in which these families cope with mental illness.

REASONS FOR GRIEF

Imagine that your spouse suddenly accused you of poisoning the family's dinner, that your teenage child responded to imaginary voices by threatening you with a knife, or that you received a telephone call informing you that the police had picked up your sister for walking naked in the street. Events like these—typical of the onset of psychosis—herald the beginning of a frightening sequence of changes that may transform a once-familiar and intimate person into an unpredictable, accusatory, and emotionally unavailable stranger. You have, in some sense, lost the person you knew, and, when the illness is permanent, the loss can be felt as profoundly as that person's death would be.

Loss of a Future

Severely mentally ill people may be impaired in ways that make it impossible for them to handle critical adult roles. A brilliant young high-school student who develops schizophrenia becomes a college dropout who is unable to retain a simple job. A housewife with uncontrolled manic-depressive illness can no longer function as the caretaker of her children. A musician is forced to give up his career because the psychiatric medications he urgently needs interfere with his fine motor coordination. Families grieve over the loss of potential—the death of a future.

The Person's Rejection of Others

Severely mentally ill persons may reject their families and friends. Paranoid ideas of being harmed, feelings of hopelessness about the future, and an unwillingness to accept help may all contribute to this rejection. One patient insisted that the mother who came to see him during visiting hours was an impostor. Another would barricade himself in his apartment and refuse to let anyone in. It is difficult, if not impossible, for those who are intimately involved with such people not to feel hurt by their hostility.

The Family's Rejection of the Mentally Ill Person

Family members may find themselves increasingly unable to manage a mentally ill family member. They become afraid to have friends in their homes because of the member's unpredictability, and are afraid to go out and leave the person alone. As family life becomes more restricted, families are often torn between feelings of guilt and obligation, on the one hand, and feelings of being trapped and overwhelmed, on the other. Members of one family expressed their ambivalence by refusing to take their relative home from the hospital but simultaneously refusing to help commit the person for long-term psychiatric treatment. Another family would insist that the hospital staff find new living quarters for their relative and then would take her home within weeks of her arrival at her new placement. No matter what action the family takes, there is no peace of mind. Families live either with the disruption of severe mental illness or with their guilt at having given up a felt responsibility.

Death

Persons with severe psychiatric illness are at greater risk of death. They tend to develop medical illnesses more frequently and succumb to them more easily. Moreover, suicide is a significant possibility for many. The family may see suicide as the ultimate statement of rejection, as well as proof of the failure of their efforts to help. One woman shot herself to death on the day her father's second wife gave birth to a baby. Another woman who had moved away from home went to her mother's apartment to commit suicide in the mother's presence. The mother grabbed her daughter's leg as she leaped out of the window, but the daughter slipped out of her hands and fell to her death. The hostility and despair expressed by patients who kill themselves may leave families devastated.

HOW FAMILIES DEAL WITH MENTAL ILLNESS

How do families cope with their feelings, and what is the role of mental-health professionals? This area has undergone a radical transformation in the past decade. Theories that place the blame for mental illness on the dynamics of family interaction have largely been discredited. Families are now recognized as an essential ally in the management of those with chronic mental illness. Perhaps mental-health professionals were humbled by the consequences of the de-institutionalization movement, which left them struggling to manage patients in community settings. Once the staff became dependent on having the family take the patient home, they had to think of something more to do with families than criticize them. At the same time, once families understood that severely ill relatives would not be permanently taken off their hands, they were less willing to put up with the criticism of the mental-health professions. Of course, there were other important factors, primary among which was the recognition that mental illness has a biological substrate. Whatever the reasons, families and professionals have begun to work together in several new ways.

Organizations of Family Members

Families have created their own organizations. A good example is the National Alliance for the Mentally Ill, composed largely of parents of people with schizophrenia. Organizations like this provide an avenue for constructive action, both political and personal. They help raise research funds, enhance public awareness of this dread disease, provide information about clinical management, and offer an opportunity for families to meet others who share their problems. One way to handle the sadness of facing this illness is to work toward eradicating it.

Family Therapy

Family therapy for schizophrenia and other forms of severe mental illness now focuses on helping families manage their ill relatives. Such therapy can take several forms. For example, a clinical staff may work with individual families to focus on problems specific to that household. The psychoeducational approach concentrates on offering formal education to families about the nature of mental illness, its management, course and prognosis. Multiple family groups allow for several families and therapists to work together in groups that focus on mutual support and the exchange of practical advice. It has been well demonstrated that teaching families specialized techniques for living with chronically ill members can favorably influence the course of an illness like schizophrenia (McFarlane 1983; Vaughn and Leff 1976).

The case of a mother who stayed at home to watch over her twenty-three-year-old schizophrenic son illustrates the new approach. The son sat in front of the television all day while his mother cooked his meals, washed his clothes, and looked after his every need. The situation was as unsatisfactory for the sick son as for the husband and the healthy children. The clinical staff educated the family about the nature of schizophrenia and showed them ways to help the young man function more effectively. They encouraged the family to enroll the son in a day program, which allowed the mother to begin to attend to her own needs and to those of the rest of the family. Eventually the mother resumed her career as a high-school teacher and the son began to look after his personal needs at home. As a result, the entire family felt less burdened and more satisfied with one another.

When Family Efforts Fail

Sometimes, despite all attempts, the family cannot achieve a satisfactory outcome. One family could not allow a son to live at home because he would periodically attempt to harm other family members. Another, whose daughter had left home, had to accept her neglect of hygiene and personal safety. The sick person's death may be the last loss for a family that has had to face a long series of disappointments. Death may be accompanied by feelings of relief that so troubled a person is finally at peace, or years of emotional distance may leave a family so drained that they have already finished grieving. As we professionals work more with the families of the mentally ill, we hope to be able to perceive the extent of their problems and find effective ways to ease their suffering.

REFERENCES

Walsh, M. 1985. *Schizophrenia: Straight Talk for Families and Friends.* New York: William Morrow.

McFarlane, W., ed. 1983. *Family Therapy in Schizophrenia.* New York: Guilford Press.

Vaughn, C. E. and J. P. Leff. 1976. "The Influence of Family and Social Factors on the Course of Psychiatric Illness: A Comparison of Schizophrenic with Depressed Neurotic Patients." *British Journal of Psychiatry* 129:123.

22

Grief, Death and Dementia

D. Peter Birkett

Grief has its hierarchies. When a child is dying or when a teenager is killed in an accident, caregivers' feelings are touched to the quick. We summon our every intellectual and emotional strength to help. We—and by "we" I mean any health-care professionals—can empathize strongly and share profoundly in the loss when a young person is afflicted. If a parent who has been caring for small children, or an executive at the height of a career develops a dementing illness, we tend to value that mind more highly than the fading mind of an octogenarian. The grief that surrounds the dying of the demented eighty-five-year-old is less poignant to us. This may make us careless in dealing with the families of elderly patients. We may neglect to deal with these deaths. Yet we may be able to do a great deal to help, and our actions may be even more important than they are in the other cases.

Those who deal with malignant diseases in the young have taught us the concept of anticipatory grief—grieving done before the loved one has died. A similar two-stage process of grieving can occur when an elderly patient becomes demented. Before death, the patient is first lost to dementia and, indeed, seems to cease to be human.

At the onset of dementia, it is tempting to physicians to try to save time by interviewing all of the family members together. Often this does not work, one reason for which is another aspect of the hierarchy of grief. Families' feelings about the loss of a relatively young member are different from those that surround the loss of an elderly patient, however well loved. In addition, the responses of family members frequently differ. Even siblings may vary much in the intensity of their feelings. Within the care facility, mundane matters such as the spatial arrangement of corridors and nursing stations can dictate how the family becomes grouped for an interview, and should be given careful consideration. Ideally, the physician would interview each relative separately but, at the very least, spouses and children should be seen separately. When an elderly patient is married, it is important to ascertain whether or not the spouse is also demented.

At this early stage, the family may exert pressure for a prognosis. "How long can she go on like this?" "How long will she live?" "Will she get worse?" are questions asked. There are considerable difficulties in giving exact replies to these questions, but that does not mean that we should give no replies at all. Families are not asking for exact information or figures.

The practitioner should be familiar with the data on prognosis and survival after the onset of dementia. However, it is surprising how scant such information is, a fact that probably reflects past neglect of the subject. Obtaining such data would seem to be an easy enough project. One large population survey of elderly patients in New York and London found that at one-year follow-up there was no greater mortality among subjects with dementia than without it (Gurland et al. 1983). Christie (1985) has written a useful review of this subject.

The prognosis for patients who have had cerebral infarcts is probably the same as that for stroke survivors in general. Arterial disease and its prognosis are relatively easy for lay people to understand. About half of the dementia seen in institutional practice is caused by arterial disease (Birkett 1982). These patients may die suddenly from the effects of disease of the arteries to the heart or brain. They tend to have generalized artery disease (Birkett and Roskin 1982); are liable to have peripheral vascular disease and macular degeneration in the eyes; and may have a heart attack in association with a second stroke.

Such things can be explained to lay people fairly simply, and the explanations are worth giving. Measures to prevent second strokes and the progression of heart disease can and should be discussed. Preventing second strokes is of course important because strokes are crippling. Surely it is better for a patient to be ambulatory and demented than to be hemiplegic and demented. (Given the nature of our health care system, the family sometimes has an easier time dealing with a hemiplegic demented patient than with a fully ambulatory one, but that is another matter.)

After the onset of dementia, we tend to assume that there will be a stabilization of grief until the onset of death itself. These assumptions are intuitive and have not, as far as I know, been tested by experimental work. One observation that tends to support this assumption is often made when demented patients are institutionalized. When the patient arries at the long-term care facility, there is a flurry of family activity. Relatives and friends visit a lot and perhaps criticize a lot. They want to know details about the food, the laundry, nursing, dental care, and so forth. A question often head at this stage is, "You will call us, won't you, if there is any change?" And then the relatives apparently fade away. We do not see much of them for a while. Sometimes it will seem, especially to doctors, administrators, and those who work the day shift that they have stopped visiting. It may come as a surprise, then, when an aide reports "Oh, yes, they do come. Every night at eight o'clock." At this stage one may neglect the patient, not in a physical sense, but in that one may have forgotten the presence of a concerned family. Then the practitioner is taken unaware when an indignant daughter wants to know why she was not called when her mother had a fever or a bedsore. The family has not faded away. It was just our assumption that their caring had worn out, that their grief had become quiescent when, in fact, it may simply have stabilized.

What indications of change should we look for in these patients? What are the indications that death is approaching? There may, of course, be fatal intercurrent disease. These patients (even those who are "young Alzheimer's patients") are in the cancer age group. A problem here is that even simple physical examination can be difficult, quite aside from the ethics of doing elaborate, intrusive investigations. Blood tests may be easier to do than physical examinations. Sometimes one does a routine screening blood test, discovers a hemoglobin in single digits, and is chagrined to find that the patient has a carcinoma that should have been clinically obvious if a complete physical examination had been done.

It is sometimes hard to be conscientious about physically examining dirty, incontinent, violent, uncooperative patients, although it must also be said that not all of the demented are in this condition. Other factors can lead to this kind of neglect. For example, the absence of coherent physical complaints robs us of the ability to focus on "where it hurts." Furthermore, the institutional settings are often places where doctors work in professional isolation, without supervision or peer-group interaction.

Diagnosing intercurrent illness in the demented is, all excuses aside, important and necessary. Knowing about the physical illness provides knowledge to be shared with the family. Then one can give them the call that says, "Your mother has a lump in her breast," or "She has cancer of the uterus." Then the matter can be discussed early. This is helpful whether or not the ultimate decision is for aggressive treatment.

Even without specific intercurrent disease, and even in the absence of brain infarcts, the patient with senile dementia of the Alzheimer type eventually starts to die. When does this happen and why does it happen? Here I have to speak from my own experience, which has only been documented to a limited extent (Birkett 1973), and the experience of the nurses who have taught me.

Toward the end (although sometimes more than a year before), these patients get off their feet. Without any specific set of causative neurological signs, without any local lesion, without orthopedic or podiatric problems, and with good physiotherapy and nursing care, they cease to walk. It may be that they just no longer want to walk. When assisted to their feet, it is as though they have forgotten how to put one foot in front of the other. This observation is not meant to condone carelessness about loss of ambulation in the elderly. Many a fractured hip has not been examined radiographically because the patient did not complain of pain. There are hospitals that are accredited by the Joint Commission of Accreditation of Hospitals where elderly patients are put in restraints to stop them from walking around. Nevertheless, immobility can occur with nothing but Alzheimer's disease to account for it. I have, at the time of writing, three non-ambulatory patients with Alzheimer's disease who have been that way for six months or more. I have told their families that these patients will probably die within the next twelve months.

Closer to the end there are other harbingers of death, such as difficulty swallowing, episodes of irregular breathing, and unexplained fevers. Of course, how far one investigates before deciding that a fever is "unexplained" is a matter more of art than science. Many "explanations" of fevers in the elderly are dubious. Bacteriuria and pulmonary infiltrates may come and go with or without fever, and with or without treatment.

Feeding difficulties and respiratory difficulties increase. Often there is weight loss. In the later stages of Alzheimer's disease this weight loss can cause tensions between nursing and medical staff and the patient's family. There are indications that such weight loss occurs independent of food intake. In practice, the family is able to say that the patient is not being fed properly, while the nursing staff say that the patient is eating well. It is important to be careful about using such labels as "malnutrition" or "dehydration." Sometimes, when families want the patient to be hospitalized, these labels are used to justify hospital admission. It must be remembered that these are potentially pejorative labels.

Autopsies on arteriosclerosis patients may reveal that they have had heart attacks, strokes, and other consequences of vascular diseases. In Alzheimer's disease, the cause of death is usually pneumonia, although autopsies produce a quota of humbling surprises. Things are revealed that should have been obvious, such as peritonitis due to perforated viscera, or pulmonary tuberculosis. Doctors who avoid such surprises are doctors who avoid obtaining autopsies.

Typically, however, pneumonia is the cause of death for patients who have Alzheimer's disease. This pneumonia is usually not diagnosed before the patient's death. What are its signs and symptoms? Its first sign is that the patient "looks ill." Quite often, when a chest radiograph is done because of this vague condition of looking ill, an infiltrate is found. Sometimes there is no infiltrate, no fever, no sputum, and no leukocytosis and yet, at autopsy, there is pneumonia. The infiltrate may become evident on a second chest radiograph, if having it done is worth the bother (a phrase that raises questions I will avoid at this point). Rapid breathing is also an indication of pneumonia, but fever may be conspicuous by its absence, especially in the early stages of terminal pneumonia.

When there are signs of pneumonia, it is time to telephone the family. Families want to be warned that death is imminent. Health-care professionals may not always appreciate the importance of this. Emotional considerations aside, there is a lot for families to do at this point. Work and vacation trips may have to be rescheduled, other relatives summoned to the bedside, and funeral arrangements considered. Even if the diagnosis is not precise, the call, especially from the doctor, that says simply, "she is not looking well," will earn gratitude.

Later comes irregular breathing, sometimes in the classical Cheyne-Stokes pattern and sometimes simply irregular. Fever may supervene. When fever, irregular breathing, and deepening coma arrive, death is imminent. There is sometimes a problem is estimating the level of consciousness of severely demented patients, who are already unable to talk or respond to speech, but at the end stage I am describing, coma is deep and unequivocal.

There is an intuitive element in the ability to prognosticate death. Those with much experience will often be able to say that the patient will be dead by morning without being able to say exactly why they can say it. It is a useful ability, and one that helps the families of patients.

In this end-stage of Alzheimer's disease, the question may arise of transferring the patient to more intensive care. Is there really any specific treatment not available in the long-term care facility? Probably not. There are heroic and energetic treatments for pneumonia, but their efficacy even for some other patients has not been proven. For patients with Alzheimer's disease who are at this point, hospitalization is largely a psychosocial measure. There are families who will feel that having the patient in a "regular" hospital is a guarantee that everything possible is being done even if, within the hospital, no bronchial lavage or serial blood-gas determinations are done. Nevertheless, the family's feelings have to be respected, even if they cause problems with utilization review committees.

At the end it may seem that not much has been accomplished by all of the hard and undramatic work, but this is one area where the difference in quality of care given by health-care professionals becomes very apparent. Technical procedures are stereotyped and can be done correctly by anyone with adequate formal training. Death and dementia, however, make demands that call forth our deeper resources.

REFERENCES

Birkett, D. P. and A. Roskin. 1982. "Arteriosclerosis Infarcts and Dementia." *Journal of the American Geriatric Society* 30(4):261-266.

Christie, A. 1985. "Survival in Dementia." In *Recent Advances in Psychogeriatrics.* Ed. T. Aried. London, Eng: Churchill Livingstone, pp. 33-43.

Gurland, B. et al. 1983. *The Mind and Mood of Aging.* New York: Haworth Press.

23

Support Groups for Family Caregivers of the Demented Elderly

Virginia W. Barrett

Support groups for family caregivers of the demented elderly are prolif-
erating. When appropriately designed and conducted, these groups are
beneficial in providing information, problem-solving skills, and support to
enable families to care more effectively and with less stress for their demented
members. Because there is no specific treatment or rehabilitation regime for
dementia, support groups for family caregivers are a primary modality for
preventive mental health.

Support groups may be structured according to the age of their members,
relationship composition, and other factors, but the most important components are the therapeutic ones. Factors basic to the success of support groups
are accurate knowledge of dementing illness and its course, and knowledge of
and sensitivity to the family's responses and needs. Dementia is not curable and
produces progressive impairment of memory and orientation, along with
generalized deterioration in intellectual functioning and the ability to care for
oneself. As dementia progresses, the behavioral symptoms change and with
them, the family's capacity to provide care. Family members' reactions vary,
and have been described by Teusink and Mahler (1984) as being similar to reactions to the death of a family member. Because of the insidious onset of
dementia and its long, progressively downward course, families travel a rough
road to resolution or acceptance of the illness. An enormous adjustment is
required at every stage of the disease as families face escalating practical,
psychological, and social problems. Without the relief made possible by support and guidance, the increasing strain of caring for the confused person at
home can increase the likelihood of elder abuse and threaten the mental health
of the family (Beck and Phillips 1983).

FEELINGS OF FAMILY MEMBERS

In the earliest stages of dementia, when memory, especially of recent events,
is lost and personality changes become apparent, families often deny the
mental changes and excuse them or attribute them to normal aging. They may

even focus their attention on the person's remaining attributes, such as the ability to recall past events. The confusion and emotional stress that family members feel is further intensified if they see a physically healthy adult who remains that way for a long time. Even after the diagnosis of dementia is made, it may take a long time for the family to accept it. Some denial of the diagnosis and its degenerative nature is normal and allows families to buy time to deal with grief; however, when denial persists for a long time and becomes excessive or abnormal, it must be recognized as such and treated (Teusink and Mahler 1984).

Many studies have shown that dementia requires more attention by caregivers and interferes more with home and family life than any other disease that affects the elderly. As family members begin to accept the illness, they often find themselves assuming new and confusing roles. One common reaction is to become overly involved in the care of their demented member (Johnson and Catalano 1983). Some aspects of this response are normal and, in the beginning, may even be necessary for safety, financial organization, the ability to function within the community, and the maintenance of health. When over-involvement persists for a long time, however, and interferes with privacy, social life, and sleep, it is not advantageous to mental health. Furthermore, overinvolvement may provide secondary gains to caregivers, such as the admiration of others and the avoidance of other responsibilities (Teusink and Mahler 1984).

As the demented individual becomes more dependent and unable to reciprocate in the intrapersonal aspects of family life, family members may respond with anger. This anger may be associated with feelings of entrapment, isolation, and a general loss of identity. Family members may feel as abandoned by the demented person as others do on the death of a loved one (Teusink and Mahler 1984). Kapust's (1982) description of dementia as an "ongoing funeral" supports this analogy. The anger of family caregivers is normal. It is not unusual for family members to displace their anger onto health professionals who are involved in the demented person's care. Such anger becomes excessive, however when it leads to abuse, withdrawal from treatment, and further denial of the progressive, deteriorating nature of the disease.

Anger, bitterness, and resentment among members of the demented person's family can exacerbate unresolved conflicts and create new ones. Loyalties can be divided, especially when the family is already disrupted or when the primary caregiver has children to care for in addition to the elderly demented parent. When these feelings subside, feelings of guilt may surface that are associated with embarrassment, repugnance, resentment, and death wishes for the demented individual.

ROLE OF SUPPORT GROUPS

The burden of the feelings described above can be lightened by support groups that are attuned to their existence and the reasons behind them. The primary goal of such groups is to strengthen the caregivers' morale, emotional well-being, and coping skills. In the initial phase of a support group, the members tend to focus on the disease process and its symptoms. Once the members are comfortable with each other, the leaders direct the discussion to include family reactions and supportive problem-solving. The aim is to prevent normal feelings of sadness and depression from becoming overwhelming; the group provides education, inspiration, and recognition of universality of the problem (Barnes and Raskind 1981). The group leader should not overemphasize negative feelings, since they do not exist in some families, who report maintaining meaningful, although changed, relationships (Rabins 1984). Moreover, there is much to be gained from sharing successful coping experiences. As group cohesion develops, members feel that they are both the helpers and the helped as they share experiences. Often, they accept suggestions for interventions from each other more readily than from the professional group leader or counselor.

To leaders of support groups, the assessment of family reaction is as important as assessment of the disease. When family members deny the dementing illness and its progressive nature, education and careful confrontation can help them accept it and thereby allow them to plan for the future (Teusink and Mahler 1984). They can also be helped to look at what their involvement has caused them to give up (such as attention to other family members, their jobs, and their own needs), and to establish priorities. Support groups can even help families gain the confidence they may need to request assistance from other family members or agencies.

If the involvement of family caretakers is excessive but provides them with secondary gains, it may be difficult to institute change. In such cases, it can be pointed out that feelings of burden have been shown to diminish with decreased involvement and with visits to the demented person by other relatives (Zarit, Reever, and Bach-Peterson 1980); that overdoing the caring role may suppress the demented person's pursuit of independent social, daily living, and recreational activities (Reifler and Wu 1982); and that the limitations of caregivers' own activities may cause them to feel that they are bearing a heavy burden (Wilder, Teresi, and Bennett 1983).

CONCLUSION

When support groups allow members to compare and contrast experiences and reactions and to share emotional needs, many benefits are gained. Confronting anger and displacement can lead to the redirection of energies toward constructive solutions. It should be kept in mind, however, that the working out of unresolved and longstanding family problems may require additional professional counsel outside the group setting.

For the most part, support groups for family caregivers of the demented elderly provide their members with a better understanding of dementia and its course and can help them overcome their fears and avoid disappointments. The recognition that problems will occur in caring for the person with dementia can help families adjust to the ensuing changes. Finally, by concentrating on practical issues and coping strategies, support groups can help members overcome their feelings of burden that, if left untreated, can lead to retaliation, self-isolation, and other forms of maladaption.

REFERENCES

Barnes, R. F., M. A. Raskind, M. Scott, and C. Murphy. 1981. "Problems of Families Caring for Alzheimer Patients: Use of a Support Group." *Journal of the American Geriatrics Society* 19(2):80–85.

Beck, C. M. and L. R. Phillips. 1983. "The Effects That Patients Have on Their Families in a Community Care and Control Psychiatric Service: A Two-Year Follow-Up." *British Journal of Psychiatry* 114:265–274.

Johnson, C. L. and D. J. Catalano. 1983. "A Longitudinal Study of Family Supports to the Impaired Elderly." *The Gerontologist* 23(6):612–618.

Kapust, L. R. 1982. "Living with Dementia: The Ongoing Funeral." *Social Work in Health Care* 7(4):79–91.

Rabins, P. V. 1984. "Management of Dementia in the Family Context." *Psychosomatics* 25(5):369–371, 374–375.

Reifler, B. V. and S. Wu. 1982. "Managing Families of the Demented Elderly." *Journal of Family Practice* 14(6):1051-1056.

Teusink, J. P. and S. Mahler. 1984. "Helping Families Cope with Alzheimer's Disease." *Hospital and Community Psychiatry* 35(2):152–156.

Wilder, D. E., J. A. Teresi, and R. G. Bennett. 1983. "Family Burden and Dementia." In R. Mayeux and W. G. Rosen, eds. *The Dementias.* New York: Raven Press.

Zarit, S., K. E. Reever, and J. Bach-Peterson. 1980. "Relatives of the Impaired Elderly: Correlates of Feelings of Burden." *The Gerontologist* 20(6):6491–6505.

24

Approaches to Loss and Bereavement in Amyotrophic Lateral Sclerosis (ALS)

Claire F. Leach and Joel S. Delfiner

Bereavement in amyotrophic lateral sclerosis (ALS) distinctively starts with the diagnosis and is progressive and continual until death. The patient and family almost immediately anticipate death when they understand that the disease is usually fatal within two to six years without recourse to a respirator. Then they live through a series of "deaths" to the relationship as they have known it until the final break, the death of the patient. In these three phases of mourning, our professional goal is to protect healing grief from becoming distorted. We believe that our patients are best served when we anticipate the causes of pain and breakdown and intervene to help them avoid the predictable hazards and pitfalls. We try further to introduce them to activities, attitudes, and values through which loss can be partly transcended and wholesome grief can occur. In this chapter, we describe issues concerning the patient and family that arise during these three phases, together with our approaches to them, gleaned from our work at the Muscular Dystrophy Association Neuromuscular Clinic support groups for families of patients at the clinic.

ALS AND INTRINSIC LOSS

The force underlying bereavement in ALS, apart from broken relationships, is the relentless march of physical losses intrinsic to the disease. These losses are deeply corrosive of the psychic energy patient and family need to deal with the threats to their relationship. The progressive weakness of voluntary muscles, in variable order, leads to the inability to move, to ingest food or swallow saliva, to speak, and to breathe. Inexplicably, the eyes and sphincters are spared, as is the heart (an involuntary muscle). What patients perceive as intolerable depends on their pre-ALS character and life style: activities, pleasures, responsibilities, goals, and dreams. The more physical, like actor David Niven, will be more impaired than those, like U.S. Senator Jacob Javits, who have lived by their minds. The articulate woman will lose more of herself through distorted speech than will a taciturn fisherman; the young will probably feel more unbearably cheated than the old.

Nearly all patients perceive as intolerable losses the inability to express their needs, to act toward fulfilling them, to be useful, to have some freedom, to fit in physically and socially with their associates, and to be in control of their bodies. Family members, friends, and professionals commonly react in a similar way. Besides the drain on psychic energy, we see in these primary physical losses two further implications for the break in relationships. The first is the possibility that others will physically or emotionally avoid the patient who arouses such distressing feelings. The second is the belief that is frequently expressed — by the patient and others — that under the circumstances, dying and separation are not to be dreaded nearly as much as "dying by inches." In some cases, the elusiveness of death causes depression and affects decision making about the use of life-support equipment.

Thus, ALS is a disease in which loss is a central source of suffering. The disease is relatively free of pain. The treatment for it is comparatively benign. There is no ostracism attached to it because of contagion. To some, the fact that it is almost predictably time-limited is a redeeming characteristic compared to the long chronic diseases or the unpredictably recurring ones. The mind typically remains clear and the personality remains intact if the disease's emotional turmoils can be handled successfully. Typically, the death itself is peaceful.

But the losses are relentless and unremitting. Therefore, our first responsibility is to do all we can to minimize their effects. Good medical management, planned by a neurologist, is basic; it involves medication, occupational therapy, physical therapy, communication therapy, and a consulting nurse who offers guidance about the personal care of the patient at home. The patient and family need to be made aware, usually by a medical social worker, of every aspect of the social support system available to them. There are financial resources, respite services, and different levels of personal care available at home or in the community, as well as members of the extended family, friends, spiritual counselors, and support groups. In addition, there may be research or other ALS projects to which they can make their unique contribution. Patients and families need to be aware that depression and tension exaggerate the natural symptoms of ALS, including weakness, spasm, and difficulty with coordination, so that it is not weak or self-indulgent for them to seek peace of mind through professional counseling. All these aspects of their social support system tend to raise the level of psychic energy and to compensate to some extent for the losses, to make them at least easier to bear. In short, whatever serves mental health — whatever offers self-direction, purpose, enjoyment, and self-worth — contributes to assimilating the losses.

After all the external things have been done, however, we, the patients, and their families have to confront their capacity for either absorbing loss as a fact of life or for mourning constructively. It is necessary to define what we want to achieve in order to direct our efforts during the three phases of bereavement.

SOME PROFESSIONAL AIMS

Some time ago we began to identify general treatment goals for our ALS patients and their families (Leach and Kelemen 1985). Since then we have amplified and refined these goals out of our continuing professional experiences, from reading, from dialogue with colleagues on the hospice staff who work with the bereft, and from our own brushes with mortality. These goals comprise a mental checklist for us now as we initiate activity, listen a little more perceptively, or are alert to detect a patient's readiness to deal with a subject that we anticipate may become troublesome.

Regarding the Patients

Consciously or unconsciously, they are getting ready to die. What helps them reach the point at which they can let go? Our hope is that they will come through ALS with their sense of dignity and worth intact, with a sense of connectedness to their immediate world, and satisfaction with the way they have dealt with the challenge of ALS. The disease gives patients time to decide what is important to them. We want the patients to make choices that ensure that they use their time for things that are indeed important to them. We believe that people can face the end of life with greater peace of mind if they feel they have not left too many loose ends.

Linn, Dennis, and Matthew (1979) suggested seven needs that remain valid even when psychologically disengaged from their religious implications: (1) to be free of bitterness through having forgiven; (2) to have passed on treasures, either material or mental; (3) to say good-bye and to provide for those who are still living; (4) to share any fears; (5) to die where and with whom one wishes; (6) to recall and reminisce, perhaps happily; and (7) to have reached some philosophical or spiritual peace about what death means. To the extent that patients wish to make plans or to resolve unfinished business, they need unfrightened people with whom to do it. As professionals, we need to recognize the needs at which the patients hint; to be open to listen and help or refer them to other qualified professionals; and to help prepare close family members for perhaps the most valuable and intimate roles in this process.

Regarding Families

The members of patients' families are readying themselves for separation from the patient and for continuing their own lives. Our goal is for them to emerge physically well, emotionally intact, and, like the patient, satisfied with the way they have met ALS. They seem best able to accept the patient's death and their own feelings about it if they (1) have rectified matters about which they have felt guilty or resentful in their pre-ALS relationship, (2) have used the available time for things that were important to them in their relationship with the patient, (3) believe everything that could be done was done, (4) have given it their personal best, (5) have achieved some practical independence from the patient, (6) have supportive contacts with other surviving family and friends, and (7) have some coherent sense of the place of sorrow and death in human experience. Like many people, they may be content to live out their lives with a variety of feelings that might be described as symptoms of unresolved grief. They may, over time, come to terms with them in conversations with relatives, friends, or clergy or in prayer or new relationships. Without laying added burdens of apprehension or obligation on them, we consider it appropriate to identify personal points of tension that may be subject to resolution during the patient's lifetime and to initiate discussions of the points of stress that are common to nearly all patients and families who cope with ALS.

The focus is not on getting ready for death but on how the years between the diagnosis and death can be used to handle bereavement constructively, to bring life to a satisfactory close, and to enable relatives to go on living satisfactory lives. Nothing can remove the mystery of death through which the patient will go alone, nor alter the separation of beloved companions. What we, as therapists and counselors offer, is our willing presence and our implicit understanding that difficulty and even tragedy are a part of living. We offer the view that when one does not have time or energy to squander, both can take on unexpected value. Our overall emphasis is on living to the fullest; fortunately, the same qualities that enhance life tend to lead toward grieving unencumbered by bitterness, guilt, or regret.

LOSS OF THE SENSE OF THE FUTURE: ANTICIPATORY GRIEF

Anticipatory grief starts when the neurologist presents the diagnosis and its implications. The timing and tone make an appreciable difference in the degree of shock, depression, and anger experienced by the patient and family and can set the mood for the duration of the illness. The presentation is less shocking if it is handled realistically over time while tests are done, the progression of the disease is noted, and mimicking conditions are ruled out.

The patient and family ought to learn, first, that ALS is one of several neuromuscular diseases of differing severity, and then, that it is the progressive and irreversible form of paralysis. At this point the neurologist must judge how much and how soon the patient wants more information. Legally, the patient must know the probable course of the disease in order to give informed consent for treatment. Furthermore, it is our ethical responsibility to give patients information on which they may wish to base decisions. But in these early stages, nothing is lost by giving patients time to absorb the information at their own pace, and much may be gained in avoiding an indigestible emotional overload. Entrenched, intractable depression or destructive denial are real possibilities.

Three circumstances may occur in which we would withold or defer information, or share it only with family members: if the patient is physically too sick to understand (which is rare at the point of diagnosis), if the patient is demented, or if the patient is suicidal. Otherwise, we believe that ALS is properly treated as a not-quite-universally terminal disease from approximately the time of the diagnosis. However, we also offer realistic hopes at the same time: that research is underway continuously; that, in some rare and unexplained cases, people survive for ten, twenty, or thirty years; that a respirator extends life for an indefinite period; and, most important, that much is known about keeping life with ALS manageable. If patients come to the clinic with a vague idea that they have a nerve disorder, and the family, with full and accurate information, wants the patient "spared" the truth, we must learn whether the family's opinion is well based — for example that, knowing the diagnosis, the patient could not continue to function because of a history of psychiatric problems. Or we may need to give the family time to work out their anxieties before discussing the diagnosis with the patient. In any event, it is important to take the family seriously because their relationship with the patient and role in the patient's care will become increasingly significant as the patient becomes more dependent physically. Professionals should demonstrate regard for them as well as for the patient, and recognize their concern, knowledge and involvement.

When ALS and Lou Gehrig's disease are mentioned, professionals must be prepared for a new wave of emotional shock, since these names can summon up vivid mental images of loss of function and make the future appear more real than do the more formal medical words. Doctors may also need to be ready for patients' and families' displaced criticism or anger at them as the bearers of bad news that they cannot reverse. Whether or not such anger is expressed, two things need to be done at this point. Patients need to be assured of their doctors' continuing interest and ability to ameliorate symptoms, and to be enlisted as the primary partner in the management of the disease.

From the time of diagnosis the medical social worker is routinely involved in making explicit to the patient and family the process of being actively involved in managing their lives, given the possibilities of each day. A redirection of hope helps forestall depression before it becomes intractable. The explicit message is that the disease is manageable. Physical dependence does not automatically mean emotional dependence. Taking care of tensions and depression may moderate the severity of the symptoms. We let the patient and family know that the social worker is concerned primarily with the influence the diagnosis may have on them and with the external and internal resources that will be useful to them.

We take a psychosocial history, explaining directly to patients that we want to be acquainted with them so that we will have a starting point if something comes up in which they would like our participation. If their anxieties have already surfaced, we may arrange two or three counseling sessions or a specialized referral. If they are absorbing this new experience with family or religious supports or are still too immobilized to know what worries them, they are told that the social worker will see them when they come to the clinic. The implicit message is that life is going on with them in charge and that experienced personnel are standing by to assist them in a number of known ways.

We understand that disbelief, shock, depression, and, perhaps, outrage and a sense of betrayal will need to run their course and find expression. We believe that the course of anticipatory grief will be shorter and less debilitating if the prospect of a difficult disease and impending death has been at least challenged by realistic hope. Many choices will remain within patients' control, and they may discover unanticipated growth and satisfactions.

GRADUAL LOSS OF THE FAMILIAR RELATIONSHIP

A second sort of bereavement occurs between the knowledge that death will come and the patient's actual death. The family and patient may come to feel that they are losing, or have lost, much of the person they have known. Both watch the patient die gradually, the process punctuated by pronounced life-changing losses of function. The erosion of the patient's ability to fulfill his or her customary roles and to perform characteristic activities is visible. In our action-oriented Western society, we often equate people's essence with their occupation. Therefore, we try to introduce early and to reinforce, whenever appropriate, the concept that people are more than the sum of their activities. We bring to attention the patient's innate qualities and manifestations of kindness, patience, and interest in other people, as well as the qualities that may not be helpful but are characteristic of the person regardless of his or her physical capacity. Thus, patients remain real, functioning individuals who bring their own influence to bear and to whom their families can respond.

Because the appreciation of qualities rather than achievements may involve a rethinking of values, we encourage the patient and family to look at the societal, familial, and personal assumptions, often unconscious, that have governed their activities. By so doing, they may be better able to see what is applicable in their new and continually changing situations. We may direct their thinking toward values that other people have found resistive to bereavement: deepened relationships; integrity in choosing one's own way of meeting an adversary; faith; and challenging some of society's emphasis on competition, measurable achievement, and conformity. We suggest that they look at what matters to them in their relationships and understand that they may grieve for lost possibilities. They may also discover closeness in the way they appreciate each other or live together satisfactorily in the face of a shared and unparalleled problem.

Communication

In this phase of loss, the exchange of thoughts and feelings that is central to most vital relationships may be impoverished physically or emotionally. If the difficulty is physical, we introduce alternative means of communication by way of speech pathologists who are familiar with ALS. These alternatives range from speech exercises to sophisticated computers with display, printout, and voice capabilities that are usable if the patient has any muscle that is capable of even an eighth of an inch of movement. Here, as with all devices, we may try to mediate between the family's impatience in trying to understand and the patient's reluctance to acknowledge a new loss by agreeing to use a communication device. We also point out the therapeutic value of body language.

When the diminished exchange is due to emotional causes, we explore the family's pre-ALS patterns of communication. In a joint interview, family members may come to see how isolated and alone each one has felt, and give conscious attention to each other's style of opening up about difficult subjects. Regardless of their earlier patterns, we do not equivocate about the importance of communication in this situation. If there is basic trust in the relationship, even noncommunicators can learn to share to some degree and not merely assume what is on their partner's mind. We introduce techniques for opening up communication, while giving each person room for solitude. If they need and want it, we refer them for ongoing communication therapy or provide it ourselves.

The Patient's Withdrawal from Family Life

The relationship may also be diminished by the patient's withdrawal from participation in family life. The patient may do so because of a fear-filled self-absorption, resentment of the mobility of others, or preoccupation with an agenda that the patient feels the family would not listen to. Such withdrawal often stems from a lowered sense of self-esteem and usefulness, and from guilt at being a burden: "I am no longer worth listening to." Consequently, we try to help the patient and family understand the patient's continuing autonomy and psychological self-reliance and recognize that these can be durable *if they are expected to be, and if they are nurtured, sustained, and actively promoted.* The patient's interest, judgment, opinion, and expertise in family matters can be solicited and remain valuable. Not soliciting them may encourage the patient to retreat and become unnecessarily dependent and so foster resentment in the caregiver. Equally, the family should be ready to listen to the patient's interests, goals, fears, and discoveries, even though these may include plans for dying. We point out that the patient and family can move past many disheartening feelings, given a chance to experience, express, and resolve them, and that this is part of normal grieving.

Protective families, meaning well, may exclude patients out of a desire to spare them added responsibility or worry. A family may also sometimes exclude a patient in their own (probably unconscious) effort to prepare for the time when the patient will no longer be there. This type of exclusion may be addressed in the supportive and less personal atmosphere of a group or within a well-established therapeutic relationship, but not usually on an educational, cognitive level.

Break in the Relationship

Infrequently, an outright break in the relationship occurs before the patient's death. We have observed this when the primary caregiver has an ego so fragile as to be overwhelmed by the physical and emotional stresses of ALS; when the relationship has existed in name only for many years (although the relative may stay on as the caregiver); or when either the patient or the caregiver displaces resentment of the circumstances onto the other so that hostility escalates. It may also occur when patient and caregiver become involved in a destructive power struggle, in which the patient uses the power of his or her real needs to exact immediate care and services as a means of domination, and the caregiver uses his or her real physical control over the patient's well-being as a means of reward, punishment, and domination. Such power struggles may be responsive to psychotherapy if the participants will use it (they never have, in our experience), or the adversaries may go through the course of the disease in bitter unhappiness. Displacement of anger and small power struggles, which are common, are usually responsive to cognitive insight if the basic relationship is a loving one.

As early as possible, we try to identify the individual pre-ALS factors that contribute to pain and breakdown during the more demanding days of the disease. We recommend specialized psychotherapeutic care while there is still some relationship within which the family can maneuver. We no longer overlook simmering conflicts within the family, even when they are not presented as immediate problems — for example, conflict between adult children and a patient's second spouse; disagreement over the proper care of a disabled adult child of a patient; marital discord; and potentially competing needs for limited material resources. We try to help the patient and family anticipate and use their option for preventive action if they wish to do so.

Some problems in relationships occur in response to the disease. Its losses, its disruption of income and roles, and the intensified interdependence of the patient and primary caregiver exaggerate things that were passing irritations when both parties had the physical and emotional latitude to sidestep them or to fight back. This kind of problem is often ameliorated if the participants recognize ALS's measured future; are cognitively aware of common psychological responses such as projection, displacement, and anticipatory grief; and use various behavioral coping techniques such as living a day at a time, learning healthy assertiveness techniques, and choosing useful attitudes. Education and information that demystify the disease and teach physical ways of handling it strengthen the patient's and family's confidence, security, and mastery. Helping family members recognize and meet their own needs removes later reasons for resentment, frees the patient from living with a martyr, and tends to maintain a two-way relationship. Encouraging the patient and family (to the extent of their ability, with or without professional help) to confront the inevitable emotional turmoils as they arise helps to resolve conflicts and enables them to move on. Here, again, the advantage is twofold; it allows for a richer present relationship and minimizes questions and regrets that might later plague a dying patient or surviving family member.

Our conduits for this combination of treatment techniques include dependable scheduled medical appointments every two to three months; the availability of the professionals by telephone; family support groups moderated by the medical social worker, with the neurologist attending selected sessions; and individual and family counseling with the medical social worker. We make use of specialized referrals, when indicated, for marriage counseling, child guidance, sex therapy, or spiritual counseling. It is our clinical impression that our intervention in potential psychological losses decreases the impact of the inherent physical loss and bereavement.

Disruptions in Other Relationships

Other disruptions in relationships may compound the experience of loss. Some extended family members and friends may avoid contact because of sadness, horror, over-identification with the patient, loss of the only basis for the relationship, or simply because they do not know how to behave or what to say. The family can sometimes modify such disruptions by letting others know how they could be of help. The patient sometimes perceives the general public to be unkind or disdainful. We accept their feeling of being conspicuous and may follow it up with some questions: Do others really feel that way? How much do you want to do the things that bring you to pulic attention? How much does the anonymous public matter to you? Does your attitude toward your limitations affect other people's attitudes?

Regrettably, professionals also may retreat, putting distance between themselves and someone who makes them feel helpless and hopeless. Families and patients sometimes surmount their hurt and anger by their perceptive insight into this professional syndrome. The antidote for the professionals clearly is competence in providing palliative care and emotional support, and a set of values that acknowledges these as worthwhile goals.

LIFE ON A RESPIRATOR

A special form of bereavement may occur if the patient chooses life on a respirator. Death is indefinitely postponed, but communication, short of that made possible by the use of sophisticated computers, is lost. The family anxiously tries to understand, anticipate, meet needs, and reach out to the patient, who cannot initiate a contact and can respond, if at all, only with signals for yes and no. With an elderly, totally paralyzed patient who has been on a respirator for many months, it can be difficult to tell if she is mentally and emotionally intact. The sense of loss and separation is probably greater for family members under these circumstances than is the patient's actual death. We can only guess, appalled, at what the implications for lost relationships may be for the patient. Thus, the use of a respirator is emotionaly tolerable only after the patient and family make a clear, vividly informed decision that this is what the patient wants and that the family can manage.

For the fortunate few who are able to use the computer, the picture may change completely. Communication, contact, human exchange, and humor can be preserved, and for some (though not all), this makes all the difference about whether life is worth living. Broken relationships at least are no longer the issue.

LOSS OF LIFE

If the patient decides against a respirator, the most fundamental preventive mental-health principle is to encourage a clear decision by the patient, and comprehension by the family, that the patient wants the disease only to run its natural course. In addition, hospital and legal rules must be clarified in order to guarantee that the patient's wishes will be respected.

In the unhappy circumstance in which breathing muscles sustain life while communication and all other mobility are gone (except eye and sphincter control), it is small wonder that some patients and families consider death to be a better alternative. We offer any appropriate palliative measures, but the principle sustaining intervention is to stand by and not to abandon them in this extremity. We can, with integrity, ease the patient's and family's guilt about their wish for the patient's death by assuring them that such wishes are understandable and natural.

More commonly, breathing fails while some other functions remain. In this case, both the patients and their families may fear a choking, smothering struggle. We can reduce the trauma of the last days by giving them advance knowledge that the death is usually calm (because carbon dioxide narcosis increases drowsiness), and by ensuring that palliative measures, also discussed ahead of time, are put into place. More reassuring than our professional descriptions are the reports of members of our family support group, which confirm our description. It is common for group members to add that the time was rewarding for them because they were able to comfort their ALS patients and enable them to die as they wished. With death imminent, skilled and compassionate spiritual counselors may afford the greatest solace to some patients and families.

THE SURVIVING FAMILY

After the patient's death, family members predictably have differing needs. The long, demanding time as caregivers sometimes leaves them physically depleted and in need of physical rest and medical care. Psychologically, it often takes them time to let go of ALS as the ever-present demand around which their lives are organized, and they often work this out through constructive work on behalf of other ALS patients and families. The prolonged period of caregiving and the expectation of death usually mean that the bereft have done considerable anticipatory mourning. They have had to make many physical adjustments and assume many responsibilities as the patient's abilities declined. Much of the grief work has already been done, as has much of the process of becoming independent of the patient. If we have been able to do our job of anticipating the causes of unhealthy mourning and the family has responded, then anger, guilt, regret, and resentments have, to a large extent, been confronted and resolved.

Those families who have absorbed the reality of the patient's disease see death as a release for the patient and, with reassurance, for themselves as well. Some may want a few individual interviews to put their changed circumstance into perspective. Some want to round out their contact with the support group by a visit or two; the group members also want them to do so as part of their own preparation for the future and as part of their caring for each other. As time goes on, however, the different emotional issues of the bereaved are better met outside of the group. Sometimes they want condolence and recognition from the professionals to whom they have felt close and may feel rejected by the professionals' apparent indifference to them once the patient is not their concern. We make an effort to be in touch for a period after the patient's death and to acquaint the survivors with bereavement groups in their area. However, we understand that some family members want to restore their sense of the patient when he or she was well by distancing themselves from all reminders of ALS.

CONCLUSION

In addition to what are normally regarded as mental health services, anything that serves mental health contributes to ameliorating the continuous physical and emotional demands of bereavement that are characteristic of ALS. ALS patients and their families should expect us to be knowledgeable, concerned, and available. We should address their expressed needs and those problems we can anticipate from experience. We must be attentive to our own needs as well, since our unspoken attitudes and personal philosophy will influence our ability to serve them in this universal experience of loss and mortality.

REFERENCES

Leach, C. F. and J. Kelemen. 1987. "The Role of Family Groups in the ALS Support Network." In *Realities in Coping with Progressive Neuromuscular Diseases.* L. I. Charash, R. E. Lovelace, S. G. Wolf, A. H. Kutscher, D. P. Roye, and C. F. Leach. eds. Philadelphia: Charles Press, pp. 32–48.

Linn, M. J., D. Linn, and M. Linn. 1979. *Healing the Dying.* New York: Paulist Press.

Rawnsley, M. M. 1982. "Brief Psychotherapy for Persons with Recurrent Cancer: A Holistic Practice Model." *Advances in Nursing Science* 5(1):69–76.

Mann, J. 1973. *Time-Limited Psychotherapy.* Cambridge MA: Harvard University Press.

25

Therapeutic Goals in Working With Terminally Ill Patients

Irene B. Seeland

Working with terminally ill patients is not only a challenge, but also a privilege. As mental health professionals, we are called upon to bring our best therapeutic skills to a major crisis in human life—that of approaching death. This situation not only forces us to confront issues of our own mortality, but also challenges us to re-examine our usual therapeutic methods and goals in working with these patients.

Psychotherapy, as the name states, is concerned with the healing of emotional trauma, whether past or recent, and with freeing the psyche of limiting fears and patterns. The goal of therapeutic intervention is usually defined as psychological growth: greater freedom and a wider range of emotional experiences, greater competence in interpersonal skills, the ability to function well in our complex society, and the successful resolution of the developmental task of the stages of human growth as defined by Erikson (1950).

For most people, this sense of competence and a positive sense of self are closely linked to their sense of well-defined roles and identities, ranging from professional identities—whether as a plumber, nurse, clerk, or vice-president of a company—to roles in the family—head of the clan, favorite daughter, baby brother, or wife—to an identity related to their self-image—ambitious, lazy, bright, stupid, sexy, dull, pretty, poor, rich. These identities contribute to the sense of self and to the roles that people act out for others as well as for themseles.

Therapeutic work with terminally ill patients must often address a variety of difficult issues. These patients have already experienced and continue to face increasing losses of the roles, faculties, and qualities that may have been major contributors to their sense of identity. The loss of health and the impairment of physical functions, the loss of jobs and economic competence, and the change of roles within the family may have already deeply shaken their sense of self and self-worth and forced them into a process of apparent regression, rather than continued growth.

The following themes emerged over years of working with terminally ill patients in a variety of clinical settings—an oncology research unit, a hospice, general medical and surgical wards, a long-term rehabilitation facility, and private practice. Although the working environments and the duration of the therapeutic interventions varied, each case revealed recurrent themes that needed to be addressed and resolved in order for patients to achieve greater peacefulness and acceptance of the process of dying. A review of these themes may help to define some therapeutic goals in working with terminally ill patients.

GRIEVING THE LOSSES

One of the first tasks in working with terminally ill patients is to gain a clear understanding of the losses the patients have experienced and what these losses mean to them as individuals. We need also to understand patients' family and social dynamics and the roles they are playing within those dynamics. The following case is an example:

> A fifty-eight-year-old business executive was suffering from a rapidly progress-ing malignant tumor of the spinal cord, with increasing paralysis and the loss of bladder and bowel function. He had been the sole financial support as well as the emotional stronghold of his family, which consisted of his wife, a charming, passive woman, and two children, a fifteen-year-old boy and a seventeen-year-old girl. The husband had always been the one to make decisions and to support, counsel, and advise. The family had been content to let him run the show, since he was doing it so well. The father, now unable to pursue his professional role except as an occasional consultant, was unable to accept the fact of his growing physical helplessness and his need for physical care, especially in intimate bodily functions. He became demanding, angry, and critical of his wife, who felt unable to cope with his expectation that she change from her previously passive role to that of competently functioning head of the household and responsible parent of two angry and frightened adolescents. The children saw their father, who until now had lived up to their expectations of a nearly perfect role model, turn into an angry, demanding, depressed invalid, and their mother change from a charm-ing, socially active woman to an angry, frightened, involuntary nurse.
>
> The traditional family structure that had hitherto served all family members well no longer existed, and the loss of previous identities and roles left the members confused, frightened, angry, and unable to adjust to the demands of their changed reality.

This case clearly demonstrates the difficulties that arise from the effect of a terminal illness and the ensuing loss of function and definition of roles. Obviously, the therapeutic intervention in such a situation cannot be aimed primarily at restoring the family system to its previous existence. Instead, intervention must aim toward adjustment and the willingness to accept painful change and real losses. In this case, another goal of intervention was to help the mother and children develop new strengths and to help the father achieve willingness to relinquish past strengths and roles.

In such a case, the therapist is faced with the anxiety, depression, and anger that are related to the process of relinquishing. Dying patients' "depression" is often a grief that mourns the loss of who they were and no longer can be, the loss of their physical faculties and social roles, and, when death draws closer, the loss of emotional relationships and mental functions.

Anxiety and depression often seem strongest in individuals whose sense of self has been closely linked with specific identities and roles that they can no longer maintain because of the illness, as well as with a strong sense of control over the events of their lives, which they have now lost. One may find at the end of one's life that those things in which one has invested most of one's energy and time — professional or financial success, social prominence, the accumulation of wealth and property — may not be sufficient to sustain a viable sense of self when one's approaching death shows these things to be ephemeral.

When we review the losses that terminally ill patients face, the list can easily become overwhelming, ranging from the loss of physical competence to economic security to social roles and the role within the family structure. The list may include the loss of sexual function, of close emotional relationships, of control of the simplest body functions, and of freedom from discomfort and pain. Therefore, it is not surprising that patients who experience such a series of losses suffer from anxiety, depression, anger, and, at times, denial of more losses to come. The ego becomes overwhelmed with the rapid reduction of its identities and begins to shore up its defenses. What, then, is the role of the therapist in this situation?

CORE IDENTITY

The following story exemplifies a way of experiencing this reduction of identity that is different from the way illustrated by the previous case.

A forty-eight-year-old Hispanic mother of twelve childen was found to have recurrent and widely metastasized cancer two years after she had undergone a radical hysterectomy for cancer of the uterus. She was readmitted to the hospital with severe pain and vaginal bleeding and in a severely emaciated state.

Although she spoke only Spanish, communication was established through an interpreter. It became clear that she was aware of her illness and impending death. Her major concern was to ensure the future care of her children, and she spent long hours with her husband and older daughters to discuss this. She was sad but not severely depressed. She interacted in a gentle and open manner with several of her roommates, who protested strongly when the nurses suggested that she be transferred to a single room because of her strong body odor.

One day, the patient pointed to her thin arms and smiled: "See how little is left of my body? It does not look and feel like my old body any more. But in here" — she pointed to her heart — "I am always myself. Even this terrible illness cannot change that." A few days later, having said good-bye to her husband and all of her children, she died, secure in her sense of self, which seemed unaffected by the destructiveness of the disease.

Is there an inner place in each person where one's sense of self, a core identity, exists inviolate despite the changes and losses of life, including a terminal illness? What contributes to such a core identity? Does it exist in each person? Is each person aware of it or can each be made aware of it? Frankl (1984), the founder of logotherapy, described his experiences in a concentration camp, where, in the face of degradation, the loss of an external human identity, and the loss of any sense of control over fate and life, this sense of the inner self emerged in some prisoners and brought forth previously unsuspected psychological resources to help them cope with the inner and outer assaults on their persons. Near-death experiences, described by Moody (1976) and Ring (1980), often leave the survivor with a strong sense of such an essential self — a sense of core being that enables the individual to look at the vicissitudes of life with perspective and equanimity. These examples are mentioned here primarily to explore the concept of core identity. In working with the terminally ill, it may or may not be possible to help them find, underneath the various layers of roles and external identifications, this essential sense of permanent identity.

The search for a core identity can often be facilitated by helping the patient revisit significant life steps and life choices and re-experience that sense of inner purpose that may have prompted these decisions, leading to a sense of inner authenticity and meaning. Progoff (1980) had outlined this process of reviewing life choices and deriving from it a knowledge of inner purpose and meaning. Such a review may also force the patient to confront the fact that he or she has repeatedly reacted primarily to external circumstances or pressures and denied his or her inner authenticity. An experience of this core identity contributes greatly to a sense of inner peace and an ability to face with equanimity the inevitable losses and diminishments of approaching death. Erikson (1950) described the last stage of human growth as the phase of ego integrity versus despair. Having lived one's life with a sense of inner integrity, purpose, and some sense of meaning can enable us to face impending death without despair, although not without some anxiety about the unknown future and sadness about the losses.

LIFE REVIEW

In working with terminally ill patients, it has become increasingly clear to me that the conscious assessment of one's life can be an important process, one that will enable patients to resolve their individual attitudes toward the losses and anxieties about impending death. One task of the therapist, then, is to assist the patient in such a life review and evaluation if the patient has the insight and reflectiveness to do so. In this process, it is important to lay aside one's own images of what is valuable and meaningful for anyone else's life. Life tasks and purposes are distinct for each individual. Patients may derive a sense of value and accomplishment in ways that may mean little to others. The case of Richie is an example:

Richie, an eighteen-year-old Hispanic youth, had been ill with acute leukemia for nine months, six of them spent in isolation in a single room. Although he had never been told his diagnosis, he had deduced it on his own by reading the labels on his intravenous chemotherapy bottles and looking up the names in a medical dictionary. His initial depression, which had led to a psychiatric consultation, was related to his realistic feeling of having been abandoned by most of his family and to the fact that his drug-addicted brother had taken and sold all of his clothes and personal belongings during Richie's absence from home. Richie also mourned the loss of his body image as a handsome, well-built young man; he had taken much pride in his hobby of body building. He deplored the inability of most of the staff to relate to him as a person rather than as a hopeless, terminal case. Much of his depression lifted with regular human contact, greater sensitivity by the staff to his feelings of isolation, and, with that, an improved sense of self-worth. Two weeks before his death, Richie began a spontaneous review of his short life, adding up all the things he felt proud of: having stayed in school and earned good grades, not having become a drug addict like his brother, having worked after school to help his widowed mother with expenses, and having been liked, respected, and trusted on his job as an evening elevator operator and porter in an apartment building. He summarized this two-hour review with a statement that clearly showed his feeling of peace and resolve about his life: "I did not have a lot of time, but I think I did the best I could with it."

Feelings of failure and guilt over real or apparently imagined wrongdoings need to be expressed freely. It is important not to fall into an attitude of making apologies too quickly or pointing out the relativity of the wrongdoing. Guilt is a subjective experience. If shown understanding and acceptance, the patient will be better able to relinquish guilt and the self-hate that is often associated with guilt, and to find his or her own inner forgiveness.

In their life review, patients who face events that they now perceive as wrong life choices, often ones that they feel have led to a "wasted" life, will need some help in understanding the reasons for such choices and the good that may have resulted even from such apparently wrong choices. Again, it is important to allow patients to experience their inner pain and sense of failure. The therapist's acceptance of them as worthwhile persons in the present is invaluable in enabling patients to accept themselves, as the case of Joanne illustrates:

Joanne, a forty-eight-year-old housewife married to a successful business executive, was in the final stages of pancreatic cancer. She still maintained the role of a well-dressed, well-made-up woman of the world, which stood in dramatic contrast to her emaciation and her extremely swollen abdomen. One week before her death, she talked for the first time about her past life. Until then, her only apparent concerns had been to maintain an acceptable front about her illness before friends and neighbors, to present a lively and charming exterior to her eleven-year-old daughter, and to show all of the medical staff a photograph album of her beautifully decorated and cared-for suburban home. In reviewing her life, she spoke about her early experiences as a theater and drama student, her intense and difficult struggles as an aspiring actress, and the joy she found in her camaraderie with her peers. She spoke of her fear of not being talented enough to succeed as an actress without making a concerted effort, her marriage of convenience to the attractive and well-to-do business executive, the "phoniness" of her resulting life, including her beautiful home, and her lack of a sense of authentic engagement in her human relationships. She expressed her deep regrets for what she now considered to have been compromise and deplored her inability to break out of this inauthentic life because of her need for comfort and security. "In a way, I am glad that it is coming to an end. My life has been such a lie for such a long time. Now I don't have to continue to pretend any more."

"ALTER EGO"

One major goal of conventional therapy is to strengthen the patient's ego. Issues of autonomy and emotional independence are explored and are often used as guideposts by which to measure the progress of the therapy. In our work with terminally ill patients, we are often faced with people whose egos are threatened by major losses and who may be faced with accepting lower levels of functioning and greater dependence because of their physical helplessness and emotional fragility.

Some patients react with denial or counteractive behavior to offset the impact of their decline for as long as possible. Others regress to childlike dependence, with a low tolerance for frustration and demanding, clinging behavior, and labile emotions. Decision-making may become increasingly difficult for them, so that the therapist may, at times, be faced with the task of taking on the role of a parental figure and "alter ego" who lends adult strength and competence to shore up the patient's failing ego structure. The therapist may also have to function as a patient advocate to help the patient express and execute wishes that may be contrary to those of the family or other medical professionals. A major issue may be the patient's desire to sign a living will or leave specific instructions about preferred treatment.

The potential danger of this direction is clear: the therapist may take on such a role too early, which will lead the patient to greater regression and dependence than is necessary. Although taking control of another person's life is not the therapist's role, lending support and strength in time of need may well fall into the legitimate realm of the therapist who works with those who are terminally ill.

LOVE AND LAUGHTER

Expressing human care actively and explicitly in therapy is not frequently taught in schools that train psychotherapists of any professional background. Patients who are dying, who are struggling with their own sense of self-worth and identity, who are facing past failures and old guilt need to know that they are considered worthwhile by their therapist. Our own concerns about transference and countertransference, which may often legitimately occupy our thinking in regular therapy, have to be weighed against dying patients' real need to know that they are loved and cared about. The active expression of authentic caring, including physical reaching out and touching, may be essential features of effective therapeutic intervention.

> Lisa, a twelve-year-old Chinese immigrant, had undergone radical surgery for a malignant ovarian tumor. Initial hopes for her cure had to be given up after rapid recurrence of the disease following intensive chemotherapy. Lisa, although not "officially" aware of the poor prognosis of her disease, showed in her realistic adjustments of future plans that she knew that her time was limited. She established a strong and caring relationship with the staff on her ward, and after a last return home for Christmas, which was cut short by her rapid physical deterioration, she seemed content to spend the holidays with the staff. On her last day of life, she drifted in and out of sleep, holding tightly to the hands of a female cousin and a consultant psychiatrist who had visited her daily for the past six months. She once opened her eyes and asked that these two people remain with her for "a little while longer." An hour later, she released their hands and said, "It's O.K. now, now you can go." She died peacefully an hour later.

To be able to laugh in the face of overwhelming circumstances is a singularly human attribute. Dying is a task that all human beings must ultimately face. The normality of this task should be kept in mind when the "Why me?" question arises. Certain circumstances may appear especially cruel to the patient and therapist alike. They are rarely unique. It is important for the therapist to find a healthy balance between empathic understanding of the patient's emotional struggles and physical suffering and the knowledge that the patient has entered into a process that is, besides birth, the most commonly shared human experience. The case of Mr. P is an example.

> Mr. P, a sixty-seven-year-old retired schoolteacher, was admitted to a long-term care facility in an advanced stage of amyotrophic lateral sclerosis, a disease involving progressive paralysis of all motor functions. At the time of admission, the only voluntary muscle function he had left was opening and closing his eyes. Communication was established by means of a letter board on which he could painstakingly spell out words. His physical condition and dependence on a respirator precluded any involvement in social activities that would have required leaving his bed. Volunteers who came to read to him quickly became discouraged by his poor tolerance of frustration and their difficulty in accepting his physical deterioration. When it was suggested that he could choose films on videotape that he could watch, he responded enthusiastically, but he requested that volunteers be found to view the films with him. He chose films that ranged from slapstick comedy to funny soft pornography, and he and the volunteers found laughter and companionship in the shared experience.

Helping to engage the patient in the process of living and loving, of joy and laughter while dying may be one of the most essential aspects of therapeutic intervention. Even while physically dying, we can engage in life. An exclusive preoccupation with present and future losses, physical deterioration, and impending helplessness can lead to a sense of hopelessness and despair that makes the remaining time meaningless. The therapist's creativity in helping the patient realize what dimensions of life are still realistically available may make a major difference in the quality of the remaining time. The experience of Mrs. M. is a case in point:

> Mrs. M, a seventy-two-year-old married woman, was suffering considerably from metastatic bone pain secondary to breast cancer. Her seventy-nine-year-old husband took loving care of her at home, but her increased pain required her admission to the hospital for pain control. Mrs. M was depressed, preoccupied with her pain, the medication schedule, and her progressive deterioration. Although the pain was soon controlled with oral medication, she refused any discharge plans for fear of recurrent pain. Life intervened with the announcement of her granddaughter's marriage. Mrs. M accepted discharge home to participate in the wedding and remained at home awaiting the birth of her first grandchild. One month after the birth of a healthy grandson, she returned to the hospital to die, having spent twelve months at home participating in the reality of continuing life.

The therapeutic goals briefly reviewed here have been relevant in working with a variety of patients; the case vignettes offer only a few examples. It is important, however, to state clearly that these goals are not universally applicable. Various factors may militate against realization of some or any of the outlined goals, including the patient's level of self-awareness and ability to reflect, the patient's degree of willingness to face his or her past life and impending death, and overwhelming and catastrophic physical conditions. Human concern and availability, consistency of caring, and phsyical presence may be all that the therapist has to offer. In working with those who are terminally ill, we may find that these can be the most important means of bringing "healing" and comfort to those who allow us to share in their dying.

REFERENCES

Erikson, E. 1950. *Childhood and Society*. New York: W. W. Norton & Co.
Frankl, V. 1984. *Man's Search for Meaning*. New York: Simon & Schuster.
Moody, R. 1976. *Life after Life*. New York: Bantam Books.
Progoff, I. 1980. *The Practice of Process Meditation*. New York: Dialogue House Library.
Ring, K. 1980. *Life at Death*. New York: Coward, McCann & Geoghegan.

26

Death: Helping the Elderly to Cope

Sally K. Severino and Avtandil A. Papiasvili

The elderly population (persons aged sixty and over) is rapidly growing. Many elderly people have serious medical illnesses, live alone, and have no one to take personal care of them. They are at risk to develop depression, which, if serious, can require hospitalization. Unlike younger people, for whom a stigma is no longer attached to psychiatric intervention, many senior citizens feel ashamed to seek help from mental health professionals for a "deficiency" or "craziness."

The establishment of support groups in the community will become an increasingly important preventive mental health service for the elderly. Such groups offer an opportunity for persons to express their needs and fears and to learn that they can help others by sharing their experiences. Under such circumstances, elderly people who are reluctant to seek help can be reached, and many problems that might otherwise become so severe as to require psychiatric hospitalization may be alleviated. Indeed, the harmful effects of a variety of stressful life events can be mitigated by strong social support systems (Thomas, Goodwin, and Goodwin 1985).

Senior citizens' centers were originally established to fulfill the social and recreational needs of the elderly. In recent years, programs have been expanded to include health services, group and individual psychological counseling, food and housing assistance, and legal and income counseling. This article describes the preventive mental health services that can be provided through support groups. Guidelines for establishing such groups have been delineated elsewhere (Papiasvili and Severino, *in press*).

In this chapter, we describe how feelings about death affected one senior citizens' group. In so doing, we wish to underscore the importance of this issue in the lives of elderly people, the importance of focusing on feelings and reactions to death in their group psychotherapy, and the importance of teaching psychotherapists to acknowledge and understand their own feelings about death.

DEATH AND PSYCHOTHERAPY

The need for and efficacy of outpatient group therapy with geriatric patients is generally accepted. Different types of group interventions are espoused (for two comprehensive reviews of group interventions, see Berland and Poggi 1979, and Foster and Foster 1983). In addition, attention has been focused on the issue of death. When a group member dies, as frequently happens in geriatric groups, it should be discussed (Weiner, Brok, and Sandowsky 1978). Yet, as Yalom (1980) pointed out,

> Despite. . .compelling reasons, the dialogue of psychotherapy rarely includes the concept of death. Death is overlooked, and overlooked glaringly, in almost all aspects of the mental health field; theory, basic and clinical research, clincial reports, and all forms of clinical practice. The only exception lies in the area in which death cannot be ignored—the care of the dying patient.

The "compelling reasons" to which Yalom refers derive from the literature on anxiety about death that he summarized (1980):

> Studies indicate a lack of overt death anxiety in the normal age population. . . . Several researchers have. . .attempted to study unconscious concerns about death. Feifel and his associates have defined three levels of concern: (1) conscious (measured by scoring the response to the question, "Are you afraid of your own death?"); (2) fantasy (measured by coding the positivity or negativity of responses to the directive, "What ideas or pictures come to your mind when you think about death?"); (3) below-level awareness (measured by mean reaction time to death words on a word-association test and a color-word interference test).

Death concerns varied greatly at each of these levels. Consciously, most individuals denied a fear of death. Older subjects and more religious subjects spoke of death in a positive way but showed signs of anxiety.

In an interesting experiment, Meissner (1958) demonstrated the existence of significant unconscious anxiety. He tested the galvanic skin response (GSR) of 40 Roman Catholic seminarians who were presented with a series of fifty words: thirty neutral terms and twenty death-symbol terms (for example, *a candle burning out, a sleeping person, black, to depart, the end*). The death symbols evoked a significantly greater GSR response than did the control words.

Patients are not the only people to deny their fear of death. Therapists are often not prepared to hear death concerns. "Denial plays a central role in a therapist's selective inattention to death in therapy," Yalom (1980) noted.

THE SENIOR CITIZENS' GROUP

The group consisted of seven members (five women and two men), ages sixty-eight to eighty-one, two therapists, a third-year resident, and a nurse known to the senior center. The patients were self-referred or referred by a nurse or other staff members. No group members were on psychotropic medicines; six had the psychiatric diagnosis of phase-of-life problem; and one was diagnosed as having primary degenerative dementia, uncomplicated. None had psychotic symptoms. Medical problems included epilepsy, asthma, congestive heart failure, hypertension, hiatus hernia, and circulatory and digestive problems. All members had at least one medical problem. At the time of writing, the group had been in existence for one year.

During the first five months, "loss" was a constant theme, usually triggered by a group event. For example, in the beginning, the group's meeting room changed several times. The insecurity of the meeting place allowed group members to express fears of losing their place of residence and of losing their physical abilities. "I cannot go any more to the less expensive supermarkets, since they are far away." The lateness of a group member led to the expression of fears of the loss of law and order in society. "Things have gotten worse lately." "Don't go out at night, you might be mugged." Members also described feelings about the loss of security in life. Members wanted the meeting-room door locked, and individuals gave detailed descriptions of the type of locks used for their apartments.

The initial turnover of group members and absenteeism led members to express concerns about losing important people in their lives and fears of abandonment. "My daughter moved out." "Children don't stay with parents any more." "My husband divorced me when I got older." "My daughter is going through a divorce." Of great importance were feelings about their loss of ability to assert themselves. "I can't fight back any more." "Often I just give in." The loss of financial security was equally important as they shared their struggles to manage on fixed social-security incomes while prices were rising. The greatest loss of all, however — the loss of their own lives — was denied as a source of fear underlying all of the other fears the members expressed.

In this context, in the fifth month of the group, one member mentioned her husband's chronic, serious illness. Neither the group members nor the therapist raised the question of the fear of death. Instead, the issue was dealt with as another aspect of the group theme of the loss of physical abilities. The woman missed one group session. When she returned, she announced that her husband had died. Her stoic attitude soon gave way to tears. Other group members were supportive and asked detailed questions that allowed her to share her grief. The members did not, however, express their own fears of losing a close person or fears of their own death. The theme was dropped in subsequent sessions, despite the two therapists' efforts to point out the avoidance.

About three weeks later, one therapist's mother died. The co-therapist told the group that the doctor was absent because of a family emergency. Neither in that session nor in subsequent sessions did anyone ask what had happened. Instead, group members strengthened their defensive denial of anxieties about loss and death. Some missed sessions. Others expressed anger through behaviors that were disruptive of the group, such as "playing cards" in an adjacent room instead of joining the group. The viability of the group thus became a central issue.

When the members were presented with the interpretation that they seemed to be denying their fear of death while simultaneously behaving in a way that would bring about part of what they feared — the death of the group — the members were freed to share their fears. This freedom was manifested in the members' efforts to bring new members and new life into the group. Even the name of the group was changed to the "Life Issues Discussion Group." Thereafter, discussion of fears of loss and fears of death were so intertwined that one always led to some mention of the other.

DISCUSSION

More than one author has remarked on the difficulty of listening to the elderly or the dying and sharing their feelings about death (Burnside 1970, Nicholi 1978). Consistent with reports in the literature, the senior citizens described in this article denied their anxieties about death. Yet, such anxiety was implied when fears of loss were expressed.

Also, as is consistent with other reports in the literature, the therapists for this group expressed difficulty in hearing death themes and in confronting the group members' resistance to acknowledging their fears. The therapists' awareness and acknowledgment of difficulties freed them to receive supervisory help both in identifying death themes and in presenting them to the group. Dealing with the death symbols early in the group process laid a foundation which allowed the group to deal with death when it actually occurred.

Bereavement is a reality in group work with the aged. The therapist's role is to be open to discussions of death at the slightest suggestion of the group members. It is important for the therapist to confront his or her own fears of loss or death, as well as those of the group members. By doing so, early acknowledgment and acceptance of reality can be used as therapeutic tools.

Support groups are vital in providing a preventive mental health service. Senior citizens are offered an essential support system to deal with the most stressful event of all: death. In this way the process of grieving is facilitated, and reactive depressions may be avoided.

REFERENCES

Berland, D. I. and R. Poggi. 1979. "Expressive Group Psychotherapy with the Aging." *International Journal of Group Psychotherapy* 29:87–108.
Burnside, I. M. 1970. "Loss: A Constant Theme in Group Work with the Aged." *Hospital and Community Psychiatry* 21:173–177.
Foster, J. R. and R. P. Foster. 1983. "Group Psychotherapy with the Old and Aged." In H. I. Kaplan and B. Sadock, eds. *Comprehensive Group Psychotherapy*. Baltimore: Williams & Williams, pp. 269–278.
Meissner, W. 1958. "Affective Response to Psychoanalytic Death Symbols." *Journal of Abnormal and Social Psychology* 56:295–299.

Nicholi, A. M., Jr., ed. 1978. *The Harvard Guide to Modern Psychiatry.* Cambridge MA: Belknap Press.

Papiasvili, A. A. and S. K. Severino. "Senior Citizens Group — The Supervisory Process." *Group,* in press.

Thomas, P. D., J. M. Goodwin, and J. S. Goodwin. 1985. "Effect of Social Support on Stress-Related Changes in Cholesterol Level, Uric Acid Level, and Immune Function in an Elderly Sample." *American Journal of Psychiatry* 142:735–737.

Weiner, M. B., A. J. Brok, and A. M. Sandowsky. 1978. *Working with the Aged: Practical Approaches in the Institution and Community.* Englewood Cliffs NJ: Prentice-Hall.

Yalom, I. D. 1980. *Existential Psychotherapy.* New York: Basic Books.

27

Changing Levels of Stress in Bereavement Groups

Dorothea Hays and Helen Miles

In the early 1970s, in response to community need, we developed a bereavement group program for widows. The program, which we called First Step, was sponsored by the Nassau County (New York) Chapter of the American Red Cross. It was designed to combine bereavement theory with a crisis-intervention model introduced in the 1960s by Caplan (1961). This model proposes that the experience of people undergoing a crisis will seem less overwhelming if it can be clarified, and that these people's coping mechanisms and support systems should be changed or strengthened to meet the demands of the crisis.

Silverman (1966) pioneered an individualized widow-to-widow program in the late 1960s. Her writings and personal encouragement were helpful to us. When we started the program, we did not have models for a group approach, but we hoped that the principles of peer support would also work in a group setting, especially if we provided strong leadership.

THE GROUPS

First Step groups were made up of twelve to eighteen newly bereaved widows who were seeking an opportunity to talk about their grief experience. Each group met two hours a week for three months. One group of eighteen widows met in the afternoon; another group of eleven widows met in the evening. The ages of the afternoon group ranged from forty-two to sixty-four, with an average age of fifty-three; the ages of the evening group ranged from forty to fifty-nine, with an average age of fifty-two. At the start of the program the time of bereavement in both groups ranged from three to fourteen months, with an average bereavement period of seven months.

The major difference between the groups was that the widows in the afternoon group were homemakers, whereas the members of the evening group all had day jobs. All of the women in the afternoon group had children, some of whom were of elementary or high-school age, but most of whom had left the parental home. All the widows in the evening group had children, the majority of whom had left home; none of their children were of elementary school age.

Only one person dropped out of the evening group; none dropped out of the afternoon group. The woman who dropped out did so after the first session and is not included in the present study. Other members occasionally missed a session.

Each group had two leaders, one a health professional with skills in crisis intervention, bereavement counseling, and group work; and the other a widow who had resolved her own bereavement crisis and had received special training in our program. Often the widowed leader was also a health professional.

The group sessions followed a flexible plan in which we discussed the phases of bereavement and clarified feelings, problems, needs, special areas of stress, and helpful interventions. Group members were encouraged to comfort and support each other during group meetings as well as outside the sessions. Social bonds were often formed that lasted for many years. For instance, a follow-up study covering five years (Hays 1979-80) of ninety-five randomly selected subjects from a total of 311 widows showed that 57 percent of the women were still in touch with one or more members of their First-Step group and that the members continued to encourage and support each other in making a new life for themselves as single women. They helped each other while entering new love relationships, marriages, and educational and vocational ventures.

The effectiveness of groups is difficult to evaluate, especially when ethical considerations do not permit untreated control groups. A researcher can examine the group process as it occurs from moment to moment and from week to week; First Step leaders reviewed this process after each meeting. Each group used minutes that were read at the beginning of the next meeting. We also used evaluation forms at the conclusion of each program.

These informal and descriptive evaluations indicated that the First Step program was effective in helping to relieve the anguish of the early bereavement phases. Moreover, the women gained confidence in their ability to function adequately as single women in a couple-oriented suburban society. Participants consistently indicated that they felt much better physically and emotionally at the end of the program.

The group leaders were alert to changing stress levels in the widows' groups. High levels of tension characterized the early sessions of each new group — the time when women tended to drop out. Our five-year follow-up study showed an 18 percent drop-out rate, all of which occurred during the first three sessions. We were able to reach and interview forty of the eighty-six women who had dropped out; the most common reason given for leaving the program was that of feeling overwhelmed and depressed in the presence of so many other grieving widows. The group leaders concentrated their efforts on reducing the initial high level of stress in the groups; these strategies will be described later.

To monitor the stress levels with a measure of objectivity, we adopted the resources of another Red Cross program. The hypertension screening program Seek and Treat was developed in 1975 in the Red Cross Department of Nursing and Health Services. Hypertension increases the risks of various diseases, such as stroke and heart disease. Stress seems to cause increased secretion of adrenalin and excitation of the sympathetic nervous system, both of which constrict the blood vessels, resulting in increased blood pressure (Eyer 1979). Therefore, blood pressure readings seem to be a reliable indicator of levels of stress.

To monitor the stress levels in the First Step program and to provide individualized intervention, if necessary, we measured the blood pressure of all twenty-nine participants in two First Step groups after each two-hour session during the three months of the program.

The women were not only willing to participate in this study but welcomed the opportunity. They were concerned about their health because most of their husbands had died of an illness. Most of them understood that stress during the bereavement period made them more vulnerable to illness.

All blood pressure readings were taken by the nurse leaders and by other Red Cross nurse volunteeers. Immediately before the initial blood pressures were taken, each participant was asked her age, as well as what medications she was taking regularly and for what reasons. She was also asked about her own and her family's medical history regarding high blood pressure, kidney disease, and stroke. After each reading, the nurse counseled the women individually about blood pressure and gave them the opportunity to discuss, on a one-to-one basis, things they did not feel comfortable sharing with the group. Counseling included health teaching when appropriate, and recommendations for improving nutrition, rest, and sleep and seeking medical care if their blood pressure was high.

RESULTS

The results of the study yielded two sets of data. First, we looked at the blood pressures for each of the two groups for each session in order to identify trends and to correlate blood pressures to topics discussed during the meeting. Second, we compared all blood pressures taken in the beginning with those taken at the end of the program to see if there was a significant reduction in stress.

The weekly attendance is indicated in Table 1, together with the mean blood pressures for each group for each session. The data were also plotted as graphs (see Figures 1 and 2). Figure 1 shows the systolic pressures and Figure 2 the diastolic pressures for the second through the eleventh group meetings. Blood pressures were not taken during the first and last meeting of each group.

During the first meeting, participants' anxiety and stress were high because of the newness of the group experience. It would have been inappropriate to start the hypertension screening at that time. The leaders concentrated on describing the program and reducing apprehension. The twelfth or last meeting was a festive occasion, with lunch or dinner at a restaurant and no opportunity to take blood pressures.

TABLE 1

Numbers in attendance and mean blood pressures
of "First Step" group members for each session

	Attendance			Systolic pressures			Diastolic pressures		
Session	Evening group	Afternoon group	Both groups	Evening group	Afternoon group	Both groups	Evening group	Afternoon group	Both groups
2	8	16	24	138.5	133.6	135.8	80.8	81.6	81.3
3	11	14	25	138.2	136.1	137.0	82.7	81.0	81.8
4	9	13	22	132.4	137.8	135.6	77.3	80.6	79.3
5	9	12	21	143.3	140.8	141.9	81.8	82.7	82.3
6	9	13	22	140.2	134.2	136.5	81.1	81.8	81.4
7	6	13	19	130.3	129.4	129.7	78.7	76.5	77.2
8	9	14	23	131.1	131.0	131.0	76.0	80.7	78.9
9	11	15	26	137.1	124.1	129.7	80.7	79.6	79.9
10	10	13	23	135.4	124.6	129.3	79.4	78.0	78.6
11	9	16	25	131.3	126.0	127.9	77.6	74.6	75.7

The findings show a rise in mean blood pressure during the first five weeks and declining pressures during the last six weeks. For twenty-four of the twenty-nine (83 percent) of the women, both the systolic and diastolic pressures were reduced between their second and their next-to-last meetings. For twenty-six women (90 percent), systolic pressures were reduced, and for twenty-seven women (90 percent) diastolic pressures were reduced or stayed the same. For one woman, the systolic pressure alone went down with no change in the diastolic pressure; for another, the systolic pressure went down while the diastolic pressure went up. For two women, the systolic pressure went up while the diastolic pressure was not changed; and for one woman, both systolic and diastolic pressures went up.

In the afternoon group, at one or more sessions eight out of the eighteen women had blood pressures that were considered high for their age; six of these women were known hypertensives. Two women started taking antihypertensive medication during this time, which contributed to the greater reduction of blood pressures found in the afternoon group. At one or more sessions of the evening group, seven out of eleven women had blood pressures that were considered high for their age; five were known hypertensives. As far as we know, none of the women in the evening group started medication during the program.

To learn more about the fluctuations in the group members' blood pressures over the course of the bereavement program, but especially from session to session, we closely examined the content of the group discussions. We found that during the first five weeks, the women discussed their husbands' deaths; their own feelings of guilt, anger, and fear; and their experience of increased

FIGURE 1

Mean systolic blood pressure of two groups of women
who attended the first step program for widows

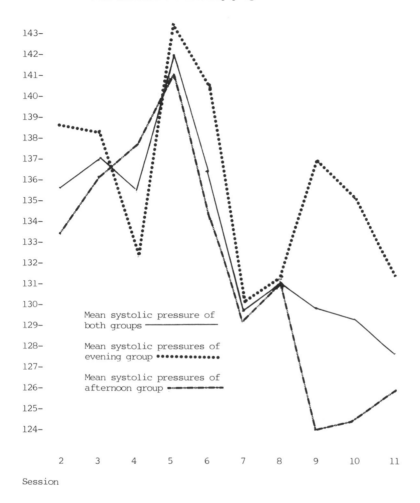

grief during holidays, weddings, anniversaries, family birthdays, and the unveiling of their husbands' gravestones. This was the time when twenty-two women (76 percent) had increased systolic pressures and twelve of the twenty-two also had increased diastolic pressures. As time went on, the women found common bonds in their shared experiences and in their attempts to cope with grief and with new responsibilities. They felt less helpless and were more responsive to and supportive of each other. Their blood pressures steadily decreased.

There is one deviation in the curve. For both groups, the systolic and diastolic pressures rose between the seventh and eighth meetings. Memorial

FIGURE 2

Mean diastolic blood pressures of two groups of women
who attended the first step program for widows

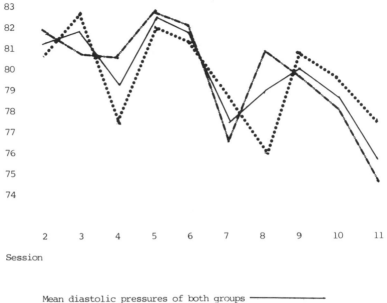

Mean diastolic pressures of both groups ————————

Mean diastolic pressures of evening group ••••••••••••••

Mean diastolic pressures of afternoon group ▬•▬•▬•▬•▬

Day was observed between these meetings, and the widows focused again
more intently on their loss. The afternoon group also missed a meeting that
week.

The study validated our observations and clarified at what point in the
groups' progress the stress was greatest. We suspected that both the painful
nature of the discussions and the initial lack of group cohesion contributed to
the stress. We therefore strengthened our interventions in both areas. First, the
group leaders worked hard to provide support and resources during the early
sessions and made themselves available to participants by phone between sessions. We also asked members in the early sessions to limit their discussions
to current problems, and either to wait to share recollections of their husbands'
illnesses and deaths until later in the program or else to do so privately with
group leaders during coffee breaks or after the meetings.

The leaders discussed and taught methods of tension reduction, including
exercise, proper nutrition, and increased human contact. The value of hope was
reinforced each time a widowed group leader presented her story of a successful coping experience. Some of us who had training in the use of relaxation

and imagery techniques used those at the end of each of the early sessions, sending participants home in a more relaxed state.

After the fifth session, the leaders could take a less central role and encourage group members to share their more painful experiences. From the sixth session on, once a group atmosphere of acceptance, understanding, and hope had been established, participants enjoyed increased benefits from the release of emotion.

To compare blood pressures at the beginning of the program with those at the end, we included only the twenty-one subjects who attended both the second and eleventh sessions. The mean systolic and diastolic pressures of these women after the second session were 137.61 and 82.57, respectively. After the eleventh session, these pressures were down to 127.71 and 75.33, respectively. A *t*-test for dependent variables yielded $t = 4.94$ for changes in systolic pressures and $t = 5.45$ for changes in diastolic pressures. Both changes are significant beyond the .001 level (see Table 2).

TABLE 2

Subjects' mean blood pressures, standard deviations
and t-tests after the second and the eleventh group sessions

Session	Systolic pressures			Diastolic pressures		
	mean	s.d.	t-value	mean	a.s.	t-value
2	137.61	17.03		82.57	7.56	
			4.94*			5.45*
11	127.71	13.21		75.33	7.62	

*significant beyond .001.

In the absence of control groups, it is not possible to draw conclusions from these data; their value is descriptive. The data show what happened to two groups of widows in a bereavement program that also offered hypertension screening and counseling.

CONCLUSION

One may hypothesize that fluctuations in blood pressure are significant indicators of stress during a group's progress. In the First Step groups, participants' stress increased during the initial discussions of painful feelings. Later, when discussions and group cohesion promoted healing and the mastery of problems, stress and blood pressures were reduced. The authors believe that the findings demonstrate the importance of monitoring blood pressures in all crisis intervention groups.

Group leaders must be sensitive to the early insecurity of group members before bonding makes mutual support possible. It is equally important that person disclosures likely to cause extreme pain should be deferred until later in the group's life, when members feel protected by a climate of mutual support. Further research is needed to test the effectiveness of strategies to reduce stress in early group sessions of bereavement programs.

REFERENCES

Caplan, G. 1961. *An Approach to Community Mental Health.* New York: Grune & Stratton.

Eyer, J. 1979. "Hypertension as a Disease of Modern Society." In C. Garfield, ed. *Stress and Survival.* St. Louis: C. V. Mosby Co., pp. 56–74.

Hays, D. 1979-80. "A Follow-Up Study of Widows Who Participated in a Red Cross Widows' Program." *PRN: The Adelphi Report.* Garden City, NY: Project for Research in Nursing, Adelphi University School of Nursing, pp. 118–137.

Silverman, P. 1966. "Services for the Widowed During the Period of Bereavement. Selected Papers of the Ninety-Third Annual Forum of the National Conference on Social Welfare." In *Social Work Practice.* New York: Columbia University Press, pp. 171–189.

PART 4

Problems of Health Professionals

28

Preventing Burnout: The Concept of Psychosocial Success

Elizabeth J. Clark

Everyone experiences stress, but burnout is a distinctive type of work-related stress. In recent years, researchers have paid increasing attention to work stress and its effects on the physical and mental health of workers. There is now agreement that work stress can have a deleterious effect on the individual worker, on job performance, and on interpersonal relationships (Cray and Cray 1977; Farber 1983; Jayarante, Chess, and Kunkel 1986; Maslach 1983; Perlman and Hartman 1982).

Maslach and Jackson (1979), who conducted some of the pioneering research, defined burnout as "a syndrome of emotional exhaustion and cynicism that frequently occurs among individuals who do 'people work'—spend considerable time in close encounters with others under conditions of chronic tension and stress." There is general agreement regarding the symptoms of burnout, which may appear in varying combinations and degrees: exhaustion, detachment, boredom and cynicism, impotence, a feeling of being unappreciated, paranoia, disorientation, psychosomatic complaints, depression, and denial of feelings (Freudenberger 1980:61).

Discussion of the phenomenon of burnout originally focused on the "helping professions" (Cherniss 1980), such as social work. This chapter addresses the problem of burnout in a subset of that group of workers. Professionals who have been identified as particularly vulnerable to burnout are those health care providers who work in hospital settings with seriously ill patients and their families. Vachon (1979) emphasized that hospice workers are also at high risk. The major identifying characteristic of these two groups with regard to burnout is the frequency of their encounters with death and grief.

STRUCTURAL FACTORS RELATED TO BURNOUT

Numerous factors can influence the development of burnout among helping professionals. These include inadequate support and inadequate training; deficiencies of the traditional biomedical approach when applied to thanatologic counseling and intervention; and lack of recognition of one's professional effectiveness.

With regard to institutional support, it is the rare program that takes into account the special needs of professionals who work primarily with patients in the terminal stage of illness. Responses to these needs may even take the form of "blaming the victim." In such cases, the attitude is "You chose to work in this area, so don't ask for any special considerations."

What is needed is structured peer support; more flexibility in scheduling; and more vacation and professional days. Also needed are supervisors who are sensitive to these problems and are willing to work to convince administrators that they must make allowances for alternative scheduling and better support mechanisms. These concerns may become especially problematic when there is only one staff person to consider, such as a designated oncology or hospice worker within a large social-work department.

Inadequate training and supervision can play a role in burnout. There are many health professionals, among them supervisors and those responsible for student training, who are untrained or poorly trained in preventive mental health and thanatology. The following is an example of poor training and inadequate supervision within the context of a caseload of terminally ill patients:

> A beginning pastoral counseling student expressed an interest in working on an oncology unit after she completed her hospital training program. As a result, she was immediately assigned a caseload of terminally ill cancer patients. Within the first two weeks, several of her patients died. When she complained about feeling depressed, the other students were not particularly sympathetic because she had indicated that she wished to gain experience with cancer patients. Her supervisor said she had better get used to dying patients if she ever intended to work on an oncology unit. The student eventually sought out an ancillary network in the hospital for support and never fully integrated into her peer group.

There are similarities in a second example:

> A graduate social-work student chose a concentration in thanatology. For her field placement, she was assigned to a medium-sized social-work department within a community hospital. She was supervised by the director of the department. The other social workers were quite happy to leave the terminally ill patients to the graduate student, and she rapidly acquired a caseload composed primarily of dying patients. Yet, during her weekly supervision conference, the director refused to review or discuss the terminally ill patients because he felt it was "too depressing." The student, therefore, was denied an opportunity to learn from analysis of her intervention activities and was also denied potentially valuable support from the director. The other social workers also had no interest in discussing her terminally ill patients with her. As a result, the student felt isolated and alienated from the department and began to question whether she had made a mistake in choosing thanatology as a specialty.

Both of these students were quickly susceptible to burnout because they lacked adequate support. Furthermore, their work in thanatology was seen as less desirable than that of their co-workers who worked with less seriously ill patients.

DEFICIENCIES OF THE BIOMEDICAL MODEL

Like others in the medical sphere, social workers are apt to see patients' death as a failure — of the health care system, of medical technology, of the health care team — and as their own failure. Internalization of personal failure and its resulting powerlessness contribute significantly to the burnout syndrome.

Only in the last few years have we begun to study "quality of life." Many of the studies done have attempted to demonstrate that the quality of a terminally ill patient's life may not warrant such aggressive medical intervention as is now technologically possible. A large literature on "death with dignity" has been developed. A major goal of the hospice movement is to help terminally ill patients live as fully as possible in whatever time they have before death occurs. Despite the research and the philosophy, however, little seems to have been written about what actually constitutes quality of life, and, as a result, it is difficult for us to know if we are succeeding in helping terminally ill patients to live fully. For this reason, it is important for professionals to discuss the value of thanatologic counseling and the need to establish goals for intervention with terminally ill patients. Particularly essential is the understanding that effectiveness should be evaluated continually, during the course of the intervention; what is occurring is a process, not just a prelude to a certain outcome.

THANATOLOGIC COUNSELING INTERVENTION

Shneidman (1978:206) emphasized that "working intensively with a dying person is different from almost any other human encounter." He also identified the different effects of psychotherapy upon the dying. Above all it must be understood that the intervention goals are different, and that the main point is to increase the dying individual's "psychological comfort." With regard to thanatologic intervention, Shneidman (1978:212) contended that "the criterion of 'effectiveness' lies in this single measure."

From this perspective, it should be apparent that outcome cannot be the measure of success because, when working with patients who are terminally ill, the result, by definition, will be the death of the patient. Instead, the measure of effectiveness must lie in the process of exchange between the professional and the patient and in the possible successes along the way. I refer to this concept as "psychosocial success," and see it as distinct from, although not always unrelated to, medical successes (or medical failures).

PSYCHOSOCIAL SUCCESSES

Psychosocial successes may be defined as the identifiable and significant events facilitated by the health professional that contribute to the emotional well-being of terminally ill patients, their families, and their friends. A corollary to this idea is that a psychosocial success should also have a positive effect on the professionals who are involved, and as a result, therefore, should help to offset burnout.

Two brief examples may help to illustrate the concept of psychosocial success.

Mrs. A, a fifty-two-year-old woman, had been diagnosed in January as having melanoma of the left axilla. She underwent surgery and had follow-up radiation therapy in February and March. In August, metastasis to the lung was discovered, and she began an aggressive course of chemotherapy. It failed to stop the spread of her disease. Mrs. A. was happily married and the mother of two daughters, one age seventeen and one who would graduate from college in December. Mrs. A was close to her children, and was particularly proud of her older daughter's academic achievements. As her disease progressed, Mrs. A realized that she was terminally ill. She maintained that her greatest desire was to live to see her daughter graduate from college. As the weeks between August and December went by, the melanoma spread through most of her left breast and it became exceedingly painful for her to move or sit up. About mid-December she was admitted to the hospital for pain control. It became apparent that Mrs. A would be unable to attend the graduation ceremony. The medical and nursing staff were doubtful that she would live even the few remaining days until the graduation. However, as is so often the case, Mrs. A did reach her goal. Although she could not attend the graduation ceremony — the college was in a nearby town — arrangements were made for her daughter to come to the hospital in her graduation gown prior to the ceremony. During the ceremony, instant photographs were taken and afterward a small party was held in Mrs. A's hospital room. The nurses and social workers who had helped make the plans and arrangements shared Mrs. A's and her family's happiness. When Mrs. A died four days later, there was sadness among the health care team, but it was somewhat tempered by their knowledge of the psychosocial success of Mrs. A's participation in her daughter's graduation and their help in bringing it about. They could not prevent Mrs. A's death, but they did contribute to her emotional well-being during her final days.

Mrs. C, a forty-eight-year-old divorced woman, discovered a lump in her right breast. She reported it to her family physician, who examined it and decided to "watch it." This "watching" continued for almost eighteen months. Finally, Mrs. C's son convinced her that she needed to obtain a second opinion, and Mrs. C. was directed to a surgeon. A biopsy revealed breast cancer, and further tests showed metastasis to the bone. Mrs. C spent eight months undergoing a combination of radiation therapy and chemotherapy, but the spread of the cancer continued. She also took a fall that resulted in a pathological fracture of her left ankle. Fear of further bone weakness and more fractures led to her to become wheelchair-bound. Mrs. C had one exceptionally close female friend, and they shared an unusual pleasure. For nineteen consecutive years, they had gone deer hunting together during the open season in December. One of Mrs. C's wishes was to go deer hunting for the twentieth year. Although Mrs. C was scheduled to be released from the hospital right before the start of the hunting season, her continuing weakened condition and her inability to walk made deer hunting appear to be an unreasonable goal. However, consultation with the friend revealed that she was more than willing to do anything possible to help make Mrs. C's wish a reality. Through combined efforts, a van was engaged for one day. The friend drove the van up into the mountains. The van had a sliding side door from which Mrs. C, seated in her wheelchair, could see into the woods and watch for deer. They shot no deer that day, but they did relive memories of the nineteen years of their friendship and had an opportunity to say good-bye to one another. The day after the hunting trip, Mrs. C was readmitted to the hospital and she died quietly two weeks later. During these weeks, she spoke frequently about the wonderful hunting trip she had had.

Other examples of psychosocial successes with terminally ill patients include events such as the patient's return to work one more time, being in a loved one's wedding, or taking one more trip to a favorite place.

On the surface, the idea of recounting psychosocial successes may seem simplistic. Most health professionals can readily identify instances in which they significantly helped a terminally ill patient to achieve a goal — one they felt especially good about. Yet, few of these successes and the roles the health professionals played in them are documented or even recognized by others. Perhaps the interventions have been overshadowed by the death of the patients — by the medical failure. It is the outcome, not the process, that is remembered. This orientation keeps professionals from seeing how effective their interventions have been. It contributes to their feeling of powerlessness to make a difference and, eventually, to burnout.

APPLICATION OF THE SUCCESS CONCEPT IN PRACTICE AND SUPERVISION

One way to use psychosocial success to offset burnout is for individual workers to compile a personal record of those events that contributed to the emotional well-being of terminally ill patients and their families, and that helped them to live more fully despite their illness. The events should be formally documented, perhaps in a log or journal format, and they must be recognized by others as effective interventions. Supervisors may wish to review workers' logs during weekly or monthly supervisory conferences. Psychosocial successes should also be presented together with problems at case conferences and psychosocial rounds.

Too often, we dwell on immediate problems and crises, neglecting to recount positive achievements. When only failures and problems are recognized, workers begin to doubt their usefulness and question whether or not their work has had meaning. Their powerlessness in the face of an adversary such as death is highlighted and their effectiveness is negated. This quickly leads to burnout.

When staff morale is low, it is useful to schedule a meeting at which *only* psychosocial successes are presented. At such meetings, supervisors should require that each person make a contribution about a successful intervention in the recent past. This will encourage workers to look critically at their work and to take note of the positive impact they can and do have. Workers who see themselves as ineffective tend to play down their accomplishments and sometimes do not even recognize them. They must be given encouragement and the opportunity to emphasize their psychosocial successes. They also need to hear from their peers and supervisors that they are making a positive difference.

CONCLUSION

Burnout is a major problem in thanatologic settings, but it is generally temporary and is usually reversible. Furthermore, it can be offset by sensitive supervisors who incorporate mechanisms to help staff deal more effectively with this potential problem. Most importantly, workers must learn not to see a patient's death as personal failure. Instead, they must be encouraged to recognize the positive aspects of their intervention. The use of the psychosocial success concept is one approach to managing and perhaps even preventing the burnout syndrome.

REFERENCES

Cherniss, C. 1980. *Staff Burnout: Job Stress in the Human Services.* Beverly Hills CA: Sage Press.

Cray, C. and M. Cray. 1977. "Stress and Strains Within the Psychiatrist's Family." *American Journal of Psychoanalysis* 37:337–341.

Farber, B. A., ed. 1983. *Stress and Burnout in the Human Services Professions.* New York: Pergamon Press.

Freudenberger, H. J. 1980. *Burn-Out: The High Cost of Achievement.* Garden City NY: Doubleday and Co.

Jayarante, S., W. Chess, and D. Kunkel. 1986. "Burnout: Its Impact on Child Welfare Workers and Their Spouses." *Social Work* 31(1):53–59.

Maslach, C. 1983. *Burnout: The Cost of Caring.* Englewood Cliffs NJ: Prentice-Hall.

Maslach, C. and S. E. Jackson. 1979. "Burned-Out Cops and Their Families." *Psychology Today* 12(12):59–62.

Perlman, B. and E. A. Hartman. 1982. "Burnout: Survey and Future Research." *Human Relations* 35:183–305.

Shneidman, E. S. 1978. "Some Aspects of Psychotherapy with Dying Patients." In C. A. Garfield, ed. *Psychosocial Care of the Dying Patient.* New York: McGraw-Hill.

Vachon, M. L. S. 1979. "Staff Stress in Care of the Terminally Ill." *Quality Review Bulletin* 251:13–17.

29

Sources of Stress for Rehabilitation Nurses

Alicia J. Goral and Florence Selder

The stress experienced by health care professionals is often related to frequent crises, the need for rapid decision making, and the fast-paced schedules of the work environment. Nurses are prime targets for on-the-job stress. In addition to its adverse effects on the nurses' physical and mental health, stress diminishes efficiency, morale, and work performance, and ultimately affects the care that patients receive. Although the nursing literature has dealt with the nature of this stress, studies have focused primarily on nurses who work in critical care settings (Caldwell and Weiner 1981, Hay and Oken 1972, Jacobsen 1978, Melia 1977, Reres 1977). More recent studies have identified stress in nurses who work in psychiatric, obstetric, and medical-surgical settings (Numerof and Abrams 1984). One area of nursing that has been omitted from such studies is the rehabilitation setting.

As the demands for rehabilitation services increase, more and more nurses will be needed in this area of patient care. Concomitantly, greater demands will be placed on nurses who are experienced in rehabilitative care.

Goral (1986) conducted a study to examine the reported stress of registered nurses in a rehabilitation setting. Eighteen subjects completed a stress inventory and participated in an in-depth interview. From the data, it was clear that the nurses who were working in rehabilitation reported work-related stress similar to that found in other settings. In addition, they reported stress arising from certain unique aspects of the rehabilitation setting.

The sources of stress identified by nurses included interpersonal relationships, concerns related to practice, and patient-care issues — sources of stress that occur in a variety of nursing care settings (Barston 1980; Caldwell and Weiner 1981; Jacobsen 1978; Numerof and Abrams 1984; Ogle 1983).

INTERPERSONAL RELATIONSHIPS

Physician–Nurse Conflicts

Such conflicts have been cited in the literature as sources of stress for nurses in various care settings (Jacobsen 1978). The specific physician–nurse conflict in the rehabilitation setting occurs with physiatrists. Physiatrists admit patients to the rehabilitation unit and are in charge of their programs. Although the nurses reported that the physiatrists provided appropriate rehabilitation management, they found that the physiatrists' lack of medical direction was a source of stress when problems not related to rehabilitation developed. The nurses' stress and frustration surfaced when the lack of medical backup for the rehabilitation patients became evident.

One nurse expressed her frustrations in this way:

> When a patient gets sick and the only person the nurse can call is the physiatrist, it puts the nurse on the line because the physiatrist only deals with rehab. If the patient needs medical management, it's usually acute, and the nurse has to [struggle] to find a doctor to see the patient. It's stressful because the patient's welfare is in balance.

Another nurse reported a major concern about backup, especially for out-of-town patients:

> A lot of our patients have medical problems that need close medical follow-up while the patient is on rehab. If the patient develops a medical problem, we should go directly to their medical doctors instead of going through the physiatrist. When the patient doesn't have a medical doctor assigned — it's usually those who transfer from another hospital or are from out of town — it's like pulling teeth to get the physiatrists to do something regarding medical management of the patient. They're too specialized, I guess.

Yet another nurse said she resented having to seek medical backup that should be readily available:

> Many times I have gone to the head nurse because I felt I had no backup from the physiatrists when there is a medical emergency. I don't feel I could call the physiatrists for proper help. Relating to a rehab issue — yes, they can and do help, but a certain medical issue that doesn't deal specifically with the rehab care — well, who can I call? It has gotten better, yet still too often, rehab patients are admitted without a medical doctor assigned to their care. Many of our rehab patients have various chronic and acute medical problems. Their status can change overnight. At times this occurs on nights when the only doctor assigned is the physiatrist. I feel I have no one to turn to, because I know right away I'm going to get put on the line. And I don't think it's my responsibility to hunt down a physician when I should be with patients. In fact, there have been times when I had to call down to the hospital emergency room to get a doctor up on the unit.

In each of these instances, one of the nurses' major concerns was the lack of medical backup for the rehabilitation patients. The physiatrists were perceived as competent but too specialized to provide the direction needed in medical emergencies.

Nurse–Nurse Personality Conflicts

These conflicts were identified as stressful by all of the nurses interviewed. Furthermore, the nurses saw conflicts with other nurses as adversely affecting the patients' care, which compounded their stress. As two respondents put it:

> Some of the nurses are not happy with their jobs. They bring their problems to work. They make you miserable because they talk about what a crummy day they're having and the crummy patients. Some of them take it out on the patients, and they take it out on you, too. It happens a lot on rehab. I don't enjoy working with those people.
> Some of the staff members that I work with are hard to get along with because they are either moody or there are a certain few that have been here longer. Granted they do know more, but the way they go about saying it isn't very nice.

Perceived Professional Evaluation

Their respondents reported that a special source of stress was their sense that they are not considered as worthy as nurses in other specialty areas. The rehabilitation nurses said that other nurses did not seem to respect them. Their lesser image created conflict and stress. The rehabilitation nurses responded to the minimization of their role with shock and hurt feelings and found it difficult to sustain a sense of self-worth. As one nurse reported:

> The disregard other nurses have for rehab nurses surprised me. There just wasn't a lot of positive regard for nurses who worked on rehab. According to some, all we do is play checkers and cards with patients. And on the other extreme, we just wipe and diaper behinds.

PRACTICE-SETTING CONCERNS

Administrative Support

A second source of stress in the practice setting is the perceived lack of support for and direction in handling a situation (Numerof 1983). In this study, nurses frequently reported that the lack of administrative support resulted in ambiguous roles and expectations. Nurses commented especially on the lack of support they perceived when they were beginning work on the rehabilitation unit. They commonly referred to "reality shock" in describing their initial days in rehabilitation. One nurse stated:

> When I started working, I kind of got thrown into it. Reality shock for real! We didn't have a preceptor at that time, so things that we didn't do a lot of in school — like tube feedings, track care — surprised me because there were quite a few patients on rehab who needed that care.

Another nurse stated:

> For sure it was your usual reality shock stuff. Things like the real patient–nurse ratio and dealing with the many others involved in rehab, the therapists and the doctors.

One nurse described the stress involved in learning policies, procedures, and organization:

> At that time, I started on the second shift with another nurse. We were short of help and were sort of thrown into the position. We had to adjust to the hospital in our new role and learn the ropes. Being a new graduate, I was used to taking care of one or two patients. Now I have five or six patients. I think I had to deal with a problem of personal organization, too.

New experiences that required them to use their judgment and to make quick decisions were stressful for new nursing graduates, as was the lack of support from the administration. Fortunately, tolerance for ambiguities is thought to increase with experience. Numerof and Abrams' (1984) findings suggest that as nurses gain experience, their levels of stress diminish. Similarly, more experienced nurses are more likely to have learned appropriate ways of handling work situations.

Patient Classification System

The implementation of diagnostic-related groups (DRGs) was acknowledged as stressful by all of the nurses who were interviewed. Although rehabilitation services have not been included in the DRG system, the nurses perceived that patients were being admitted to rehabilitation "too soon and too sick." They believed that the patients had a high incidence of complications, which retarded their rehabilitation programs. One nurse reported:

> DRGs cause stress in rehab even though rehab isn't included on their payment schedule. They do affect us. Patients admitted to us are coming from hospitals too early. When their DRGs run out, here they come, ready or not. They are coming to rehab when they aren't medically stable. We are not technically equipped or prepared to care for some of the patients, and it can be scary. I believe in early rehab, but let's have patients who can participate in their own rehab.

Several of the nurses identified a possible solution: the implementation of an improved screening process for patients entering rehabilitation in order to decrease the admission of those who are not ready for rehabilitation. It can be assumed that nurses' stress levels would be lowered if a more appropriate method of admitting rehabilitation patients were used. One nurse stated:

> I feel the doctors should screen the patients better before the patients are sent

over to rehab. I think many of them come onto the unit too soon. I think many of them come on to the unit because of the time limitations placed on the other units by DRGs. They don't know where to send them — so it's either rehab or the nursing home. So many patients slip through and come to the unit too early.

ISSUES IN THE CARE OF PATIENTS

Nature of the Population

A rehabilitation center generally admits patients with various disabilities: spinal cord injuries (paraplegia or quadriplegia), amputation of a limb or limbs, an open- or closed-head injury, a stroke, or any neuromuscular disorder. Rehabilitation nurses reported that the type of patient, the length of stay, and DRGs were sources of stress; the combination of all three of these factors is unique to the rehabilitation setting.

The primary source of stress was the type of patients admitted to rehabilitation. In particular, it was head-injured patients whom nurses repeatedly identified as being especially stressful to care for. One nurse shared her intense feeling about caring for these patients:

> It's very difficult to deal with patients with a head injury because of their behaviors. They can strike out at you. They have a terrible temper. One minute they can be as calm and placid as can be and the next minute they can turn on you. Managing the head-injured, especially the men, is really hard.

Stroke patients also may display problem behaviors. The nurses commonly identified patients with behavioral problems as being stressful bcause they feared for the patients' safety as well as for their own, and their stress increased with the threat of physical harm.

All rehabilitation patients have some problems in caring for themselves. These deficits may be total or partial, permanent or temporary. Activities of daily living (feeding, bathing, toileting, dressing, and personal grooming), which patients previously performed independently, now require physical and emotional support from the nurse and place great stress on the nurse's physical stamina. Fear of massive bodily damage and repeated reminders of the fragility of life may induce further stress.

Furthermore, patients in rehabilitation spend more time with nurses than with any other health care professionals. Rehabilitation nurses are responsible for the environment in which the patients spend most of their time, where they eat, sleep, keep their belongings, meet with family members and friends, and apply the skills they have learned in other therapies. The nusing unit is where other professionals come to visit, examine, or observe patients, and from which patients must leave for therapy appointments on time and without embarrassing problems of incontinence.

Another stress factor identified by the rehabilitation nurses was the patients' length of stay in rehabilitation. The average length of stay in an acute care setting is decreasing annually, yet the average stay for a patient in rehabilitation is approximately one month. The number of days the patient remains on the unit will most likely affect the care that is given and the quality of the nurse–patient relationship. One nurse pointed out certain personality characteristics that influence her relationships with patients. She believed that stress increases as the nurse–patient relationship deteriorates:

> Patients are here a long time. They average one month; sometimes it's a year. Patients can become very demanding. Sometimes there's a personality clash. But you have to learn to deal with it to take care of the patient. I know this is a source of stress, and sometimes the relationship just falls apart.
>
> I feel the nurse gets so involved with rehabilitation patients because they're here for so long. I know from floating to other units that a surgical patient is there for four or five days and they're gone. They're on the road to full recovery, and they just don't seem to have the problem. On rehab we tend to get more involved in the physical and emotional care of patients.

Physical Work

Work on a rehabilitation unit is described as heavy and hard. The physical workload for the rehabilitation nurse is a source of stress because it often results in frustration and physical exhaustion and, occasionally, injury.

The type of patients on a rehabilitation unit, the patients' physical dependence, the daily routine, and inadequate staffing have been identified as influencing the rehabilitation nurse's physical workload and level of stress. For instance, one nurse reported:

> The work is hard, at times stressful. All of the physical care that the typical rehab patient needs is really exhausting. The patients are often dependent for everything—turning in bed, feeding, bathing, dressing, toileting, and sometimes even blowing their noses.

Another responded:

> The work tends to be more stressful the more physical it is. And the physical stress sometimes depends on the staffing and the patient census. The more patients and the more physically dependent they are, the more draining they are.

And finally, the words of another nurse:

> We spend a lot of time with our patients. We get them up in the morning, bathe and dress them. Every patient on rehab is expected to be dressed and up. Then they go to the cafeteria, where you may need to feed them. Then you toilet them, maybe change their clothes, and things like that. While on another floor, the patients are in bed. On rehab, you have to transfer patients on and off the toilet. And if they are incontinent, we have to go through the whole process of back to bed, change their clothes, provide skin care, and still make the patient feel human.

Psychosocial Care

Another factor that contributes to nurses' stress is the continuous tension and emotional pain experienced by patients and their families. Gans (1983) posited that patients experience strong negative emotions — hate — when they are in rehabilitation settings. The patients' self-hatred and hatred of the staff and the staff's hatred of the patients and their families create a steady conflict that often results in guilt. According to Gans, staff members who work with the disabled often experience the guilt that comes from their hatred. Patients and their families are often overwhelmed in this setting; at times, the staff will also feel overwhelmed. The arousal of intense feelings and the growing attachment of the nurse, the patient, and the family can promote conflict and stress for all involved.

The rehabilitation nurses in this study did not directly report hate as a source or a result of the stress of being involved with patients and their families. Indirectly, they expressed guilt arising mainly from their failure to meet set expectations in providing high-quality care. Although the issue of hate in rehabilitation was not specifically identified in the present study, it would be inaccurate to assume that hate is not present in this setting. The rehabilitation nurses may have censored their responses because of the obvious negative connotations of hate, and an awareness that the social and professional expectations of those in a service-oriented profession militate against such an admission.

Rehabilitation patients commonly share with nurses their psychological needs and feelings about the impact of the disease or injury on them. Often they cannot express these emotions and concerns to their families. Since nurses spend so much time with the patients, it is not surprising that patients seek out the nurses to disclose their feelings. One nurse said:

> Sometimes patients just want time to talk. One patient came out to the desk in the middle of the night. I gave him a cup of coffee and then he talked to me while I was busy at the desk.

Sometimes patients use an indirect approach to express their concerns. The responsive nurse will pick up on their cues. One young woman who was diagnosed as having a chronic disease and a major physical disability was scheduled for a surgical procedure the following day. Feeling anxious and fearing the unknown, she was able indirectly to seek support from a nurse:

> She was a very sick girl, and had been on rehab a long time. I was working nights. The patient was going to have surgery the next morning. Her history was not good. She had coded [gone into cardiopulmonary arrest] during a previous surgery and the doctor had told her there was a 50 percent chance that she would code during this surgery. She was real quiet and withdrawn on evenings, and she wasn't sleeping much. I spent practically my whole night in her room. I was able to spend time with her and talk. She opened up. She talked about her family,

and said that if anything happened, she would want life support. She said she was doing that for her mother. Anyway, the patient had a chance to open up and I felt good that I could be there for her.

Family Involvement

The nurses understood that work with the rehabilitation patient meant involving the patient's family and support systems in the overall rehabilitation program. All of the nurses who were interviewed agreed that emotional support should be given to both the patient and the family. They expressed concern, however, about the problem of involving patients and families in the course of rehabilitation. One nurse said:

> Well, I knew there would be a lot of family involvement, but coming in as a new graduate I thought, "Oh, boy, families are going to want to participate in the care and to do things." Well, it doesn't work that way. I have seen so many patients who were well enough to go home if someone would only spend an hour or two each day with them. But they don't go home; they go to a nursing home.

Frustration and stress levels rise, according to the nurses, when their emotional involvement in patients' rehabilitation increases. In addition, the greater involvement of families can sometimes work to the patient's disadvantage, depending on family attitudes, expectations, and ability to work cooperatively with staff.

Regardless of the position the family takes during the rehabilitation process, the patient–family relationship is a significant factor in how the patient progresses through rehabilitation. The patient may experience role conflict while hospitalized, and the family and the patient will need to adapt to their new roles. The complexity of the nurses' involvement with patients and their families results in stress for all involved. As one nurse observed:

> I noticed, in comparing rehab to other units, that the psychological problems of patients in rehab can be overwhelming. I can sit down with patients if they want to talk, and this is when some of their problems come out, especially young quadriplegics or amputees. They not only have a physical disability, they also have a psychological problem — like dealing with body image, self-image, their problems with their families.

In providing emotional support for patients whose support systems have dissolved or failed during their hospitalization, the nurse must deal with problems that were present before the injury, as well as those that arise during hospitalization because of maladaptation to the handicap. Nurses reported cases of young patients and their families who were unable to cope with the stress of a catastrophic injury. For instance, when a quadriplegic patient's marriage dissolved, the nurses became his immediate emotional support.

Helping a patient and family cope with loss and grief requires good skills in communication and interaction to provide the necessary emotional care.

One nurse described a situation in which a patient, already grieving for the loss of a limb, was also seeking support and reassurance for his lack of progress:

> Many rehab patients, especially male patients, don't think they're progressing fast enough. They become frustrated. For example, the other night, I found an amputee patient sitting up in bed with his head down. When I asked him if something was wrong, he said, "I'm just not doing what I should be doing. I should be working faster, but therapies have been so hard on my back, and it hurts me all the time."
> These patients worry about everything they have to do the next day. They and their families are dealing with achievement and worth. We have to deal with their fears and concerns, a common one being, What happens to me if I don't improve?

The fears and anxieties patients express during rehabilitation are real. The intensity of the emotions in a rehabilitation setting compound the nurses' stress in that they must deal with the patient's and the family's emotions as well as their own.

DEATH AND DYING

The last aspect of psychosocial care is the care of someone who is dying. Numerof and Abrams (1984) reported that death-related issues are a source of stress regardless of a nurse's specialty. Garfield (1980) noted that a special burden is borne by those who work with dying patients and their families. Because rehabilitation focuses on helping patients attain an optimal level of living, rehabilitation nurses deal with death-related issues only infrequently. When they have to do so, the process can be highly stressful. The long-term nature of the relationship can add significantly to the emotional burden and the sense of personal loss when a patient dies.

One nurse stated that she felt so stressed because she felt it was like giving in to defeat after a fight well fought:

> Patients stay so long on rehab. You get to know them so well. It's so sad when they die. It doesn't even matter if the patient is at home. You know how much and how hard they worked to get to the point where they could go home.

CONCLUSION

Nurses who work in rehabilitation need help in avoiding the pitfalls involved in caring for their patients. Just as these patients and their families are often overwhelmed by their injuries, so can nurses at times also become overwhelmed in caring for them and thereby become susceptible to increased stress, resulting in burnout (Garfield 1980).

Stressful situations may vary, depending on the rehabilitation setting. In each case, it is essential to identify whatever situations or persons are the specific sources of stress for rehabilitation nurses in the work environment. The effective management of stress in a rehabilitation setting will not only improve the situation of nurses, but also ultimately influence the quality of patient care.

REFERENCES

Barston, J. 1980. "Stress Variance in Hospice Nursing." *Nursing Outlook* 28:751–754.

Caldwell, T. and Weiner, M. 1981. "Stresses and Coping in ICU Nursing." *General Hospital Psychiatry* 3:119–134.

Gans, J. 1983. "Hate in the Rehabilitation Setting." *Archives of Physical Medicine and Rehabilitation* 64:176–179.

Garfield, C. 1980. "Coping with Burn-Out." *Hospital Forum* 23(1):15.

Goral, A. J. 1986. "Sources of Stress Reported by Nurses in a Rehabilitation Setting." Unpublished master's degree thesis, Medical College of Wisconsin, Milwaukee.

Hay, O. and D. Oken. 1972. "The Psychological Stresses in the Intensive Care Nursing Unit." *Psychosomatic Medicine* 34:109–118.

Jacobsen, S. 1978. "Stressful Situations for Neonatal Intensive Care Nurses." *American Journal of Maternal-Child Nursing* 7:144–151.

Melia, K. 1977. "The Intensive Care Unit — A Stress Situation?" *Nursing Times* 72:17.

Numerof, R. 1983. *Managing Stress: A Guide for Health Professionals.* Gaithersburg MD: Aspen.

Numerof, R. and M. Abrams. 1984. "Sources of Stress Among Nurses: An Empirical Investigation." *Journal of Human Stress* 10:88–100.

Ogle, M. E. 1983. "Stages of Burnout Among Oncology Nurses in the Hospital Setting." *Oncology Nursing Forum* 10(1):31–34.

Reres, M. 1977. "Coping with Stress in the ICU and CCU." *Supervisor Nurse* 3:29.

30

Caring for Medical Students

June C. Penney

Medical students typically arrive full of enthusiasm and idealism, energy and anticipation, eager to help and to heal. They want to do the right thing and to succeed.

They also carry a burden of anxiety. For the past few years, they have been anxious about getting into medical school and about how they will cope once they are there. They realize that 50 percent of them will be in the bottom half of the class—a situation that they have never before experienced.

Medical students (41 percent of whom are women) tend to be obsessive and compulsive. During their training, they will go without sleep, eat hundreds of cafeteria meals, and give up a normal social life. They will find the work difficult and demanding: they will face a staggering amount of course material to absorb, tremendous competition, and constant fear of failure. But 97.5 percent of them *will* graduate—encumbered by a sizeable debt. Ultimately, they will probably have financial security, two children, and a station wagon. But 10 percent of them will be chronically impaired by drugs or alcohol.

It is important to recognize that in a class in which the average age is twenty-two-and-a-half years, most medical students are going through major life changes and major decisions. Many will marry and become parents during their four years in medical school.

The purpose of this chapter is to define the losses or bereavements that occur during medical education, to examine how medical schools respond to some of these, and to suggest ways to reduce their impact.

LOSSES

Medical students experience the loss of many of the elements that constitute a "normal" life: time for family and friends, time for socializing, financial security, sleep, and confidence in their abilities. In a sense, they are institutionalized for a period that may be as long as fifteen years. They also have to play the medical school "game," which requires unending competition. Typical attitudes among classmates: "I know more than you do," "I know something you don't know," and "I can study longer than you can." Unfortunately, the pressure on medical students and on physicians can lead to depression, the abuse of alcohol or drugs, and sometimes suicide.

POSSIBLE INTERVENTIONS

Medical schools do a strange thing to new students. Usually during the first few weeks, they send the students to the anatomy laboratory and expect them to begin dissecting. For many, this is their first experience of death; in fact, in a study I conducted of medical students at the Dalhousie Medical School in Halifax, Nova Scotia, it was found that 81 percent of the students had never seen a naked cadaver before entering medical school. This anonymous statistical study was carried out primarily to determine medical students' reactions to human dissection. It also provided insights into many other needs of medical students and suggested some possible interventions.

First, of the 96 percent of the students who responded to the questionnaire, 23 percent suffered from nausea, fainting, loss of appetite, sleeplessness, or nightmares during the first few weeks of dissection. Second, because of their anxieties about death, 38 percent thought more deeply about human life; 30 percent said that they saw a need to allow themselves to experience emotions so they could better relate to their patients, particularly dying patients; 21 percent said they repressed their feelings in order to be objective; 11 percent pretended that they had no anxieties; 6 percent joked about their anxieties; and 57 percent expressed to other people their anxieties about death and dissection during the course in anatomy. Third, 67 percent reported changes in attitudes after the dissecting experience, including an unwillingness to donate their bodies for dissection or for their relatives to do so; gratitude to the donors; thoughts about the death of their loved ones; and questions about life after death.

I asked the students if they thought that the anatomy department had adequately prepared them for the experience of dissection. Eighty-two percent said that they had not received enough instruction on dissecting techniques (some had never even dissected a frog); 64 percent felt that the anatomy faculty had not provided them with sufficient emotional preparation; 53 percent asked for more emotional preparation in the form of discussions on death and the opportunity to share their fears; and 12 percent requested more information on donors and burials. In short, the study found many concerns that could be addressed.

What has the Dalhousie Medical School done about the medical students' first exposure to the anatomy laboratory? It has taken the following three steps:

- During the first lecture in the course "Introduction to Anatomy," students receive information on donors and burials in the form of an information package customarily sent to prospective body donors. They are told that if they know or suspect that someone known to them has donated his or her body, they should inform the instructor and that cadaver will be withdrawn.

- Students in groups of twelve have half-hour discussions in the dissecting room with a faculty member. These discussions take place around a cadaver which is initially wrapped, but which is unwrapped early in the session. The students are encouraged to understand that the experience may be emotionally traumatic, and the anatomists tell them about their own emotional responses to dissection. Students are encouraged to talk to each other and to the faculty members about their reactions and, during the first laboratory session, to make sure that each member of the group does dissect. Discussions typically focus on students' reactions to seeing a cadaver for the first time, their previous experiences with death, their religious and ethnic backgrounds, and their concern about controlling their emotions without losing compassion for dying patients.
- At the beginning of the first dissecting laboratory, students are shown a tape that demonstrates proper dissecting techniques.

Ultimately, the students attend and participate in a memorial service for the relatives of those who have donated their bodies. A student plays the organ and another student delivers the eulogy.

The course on "Death and Dying" provides another opportunity to address some of the needs expressed in the study. This course begins with small-group discussions on facing our own mortality, a central issue each of us must attempt to confront in order to understand that death is inescapable and universal. This course also features speakers — a person who has been bereaved and a person who is suffering from a terminal illness — and the students have an opportunity to speak with them.

Another form of intervention is the student adviser program, which has been in existence for three years and which I direct. This program is confidential and is separate from the Dean's Office. Volunteer faculty members assist in counseling the students, and there is a hot line to the University Health Service. Students can come for academic help or for advice on personal difficulties and emotional problems. Another regular activity is the brown-bag lunch, at which various topics are discussed, including physician drug abuse and the rigors of coping with medical school.

ROLE MODELS

Unfortunately, scientists may be more interested in their science than in their students, and clinicians are busy people who see any student only for a brief time in his or her career. We need to take a hard look at ourselves and at our schools. It must be said, however, that many faculty members are superb role models, and many of them participate in the advisory program. Yet in fact the first role model that the medical student has for an extended period is the intern, who probably is having the toughest year of his or her life. Ought we not to consider how the lot of interns can be improved? And as faculty members, might we not stand an honest look at our own attitudes toward students?

CONCLUSION

It is apparent from the literature and from my own studies that medical students are particularly vulnerable to experiencing a high degree of stress and a sense of loss, loneliness, and inadequacy. In addition to teaching the technical skills required to practice medicine, it is incumbent upon schools to implement programs, such as those described here, that offer students the means to cope more effectively with the emotional demands of their arduous training.

INDEX